Atlas of the Facial Nerve and Related Structures

Nobutaka Yoshioka, MD, PhD
Director
Department of Craniofacial Surgery and Plastic Surgery
Tominaga Hospital
Osaka, Japan

Albert L. Rhoton, Jr., MD
R.D. Keene Family Professor and Chairman Emeritus
Department of Neurosurgery
College of Medicine
University of Florida
Gainesville, Florida

With 97 Illustrations

Thieme
New York • Stuttgart • Delhi • Rio de Janeiro

Thieme Medical Publishers, Inc.
333 Seventh Ave.
New York, NY 10001

Executive Editor: Timothy Hiscock
Managing Editor: Sarah Landis
Editorial Assistant: Nikole Connors
Senior Vice President, Editorial and Electronic Product
    Development: Cornelia Schulze
Production Editor: Barbara A. Chernow
International Production Director: Andreas Schabert
International Marketing Director: Fiona Henderson
Director of Sales, North America: Mike Roseman
International Sales Director: Louisa Turrell
Vice President, Finance and Accounts: Sarah Vanderbilt
President: Brian D. Scanlan
Compositor: Toppan Best-set Premedia Limited

Library of Congress Cataloging-in-Publication Data

Yoshioka, Nobutaka, author.
   Atlas of the facial nerve and related structures / Nobutaka
   Yoshioka, Albert L. Rhoton, Jr.
      p. ; cm.
   Includes index.
   ISBN 978-1-62623-171-9 (alk. paper)
   I. Rhoton, Albert L., 1932– , author. II. Title.
   [DNLM: 1. Facial Nerve—anatomy & histology—Atlases.
   2. Head—anatomy & histology—Atlases. 3. Neck—anatomy &
   histology—Atlases. WL 17]
   QP327
   612.9'2078—dc23   2014044551

Copyright ©2015 by Thieme Medical Publishers, Inc.
Thieme Publishers New York
333 Seventh Avenue, New York, NY 10001 USA
+1 800 782 3488, customerservice@thieme.com

Thieme Publishers Stuttgart
Rüdigerstrasse 14, 70469 Stuttgart, Germany
+49 [0]711 8931 421, customerservice@thieme.de

Thieme Publishers Delhi
A-12, Second Floor, Sector-2, Noida-201301
Uttar Pradesh, India
+91 120 45 566 00, customerservice@thieme.in

Thieme Publishers Rio, Thieme Publicações Ltda.
Argentina Building 16th floor, Ala A, 228 Praia do Botafogo
Rio de Janeiro 22250-040 Brazil
+55 21 3736-3631

Printed in China by Everbest Printing Ltd.   5 4 3 2 1

ISBN 978-1-62623-171-9

Also available as an e-book:
eISBN 978-1-62623-172-6

Important note: Medicine is an ever-changing science undergoing continual development. Research and clinical experience are continually expanding our knowledge, in particular our knowledge of proper treatment and drug therapy. Insofar as this book mentions any dosage or application, readers may rest assured that the authors, editors, and publishers have made every effort to ensure that such references are in accordance with the state of knowledge at **the time of production of the book.**

Nevertheless, this does not involve, imply, or express any guarantee or responsibility on the part of the publishers in respect to any dosage instructions and forms of applications stated in the book. **Every user is requested to examine carefully** the manufacturers' leaflets accompanying each drug and to check, if necessary in consultation with a physician or specialist, whether the dosage schedules mentioned therein or the contraindications stated by the manufacturers differ from the statements made in the present book. Such examination is particularly important with drugs thatare either rarely used or have been newly released on the market. Every dosage schedule or every form of application used is entirely at the user's own risk and responsibility. The authors and publishers request every user to report to the publishers any discrepancies or inaccuracies noticed. If errors in this work are found after publication, errata will be posted at www.thieme.com on the product description page.

Some of the product names, patents, and registered designs referred to in this book are in fact registered trademarks or proprietary names even though specific reference to this fact is not always made in the text. Therefore, the appearance of a name without designation as proprietary is not to be construed as a representation by the publisher that it is in the public domain.

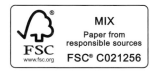

Contents

Note: Every figure shows the left side whenever the unilateral side is shown.

Preface

It has been more than ten years since I finished my fellowship at the Microneuroanatomy Laboratory at the University of Florida. I first met Dr. Albert Rhoton at the seventh meeting of the Japanese Society for Skull Base Surgery, held in Hakata, Japan, in 1995. I will never forget how deeply impressed I was by the anatomical illustrations he showed at that meeting. As every neurosurgeon now knows, his images detail delicate brain anatomy in a unique way, and it was something that I had never seen before. Then, from Septembr 2003 to August 2004, I had an opportunity to study head anatomy at his laboratory. At that time, I was a board-certified plastic surgeon and a board-certified neurosurgeon in Japan. Although I had been working exclusively as a plastic surgeon rather than as a neurosurgeon, Dr. Rhoton generously allowed me to study the anatomy of the extracranial region at his laboratory. This had been my major interest as a plastic surgeon, and I found in my research that the qualities of anatomical specimens varied greatly. For example, the quality of silicon injection of the extracranial region differed from the intracranial region, and this concerned me. Fortunately, at Dr. Rhoton's laboratory I was finally able to obtain some good specimens in which the silicon was almost perfectly injected into the extracranial region.

Facial reanimation surgery has been my life's work for more than 10 years, and with this book, Dr. Rhoton and I had as our goal the creation of an atlas of anatomy of the facial nerve illustrated with precisely dissected specimens, similar to the beautifully illustrated *Pernkopf Anatomy*. I believe that an atlas of anatomy consisting of specimens is more understandable than one with illustrations, even if they are delicately drawn. Our appreciation of basic human anatomy is not always complete, and a thorough reevaluation of the literature supplemented by detailed cadaver dissections can lead to new insights that may alter our surgical technique.

Finally, I want to express my appreciation for the patience of my children, Aya, Satoshi, Akira, and Jun, while I have been immersed in this project and clinical work. I think this book should be dedicated to the donors of the specimens shown because only their devotion made this work possible.

Nobutaka Yoshioka, MD, PhD

Preface

One of the joys of my professional career has been to work with Nobutaka Yoshioka, MD, PhD, an outstanding plastic surgeon, on this atlas. My applause and congratulations go to him for this outstanding book. Michelangelo and da Vinci and many great artists pursued cadaveric dissection as a way of achieving perfection in their art; this beautiful anatomical volume highlights Dr. Yoshioka's own passion for perfection. Dr. Yoshioka worked in our microsurgery laboratory, where he created precise and accurate dissections of the facial nerve as a guide to improving the lives of our patients. We are fortunate to have had Dr. Yoshioka in our laboratory, where he worked night and day to achieve the excellence reflected in the photographs in this book.

In sections, which begin with the skull and intracranial structures, followed by the upper, mid, and lower face and the posterolateral neck, this atlas captures the full course of the facial nerve. Each section is filled with stunning color images of his magnificent dissections, and every figure is supplemented with a concise, well-focused description that provides a wealth of information. Surgeons, particularly neurosurgeons and plastic surgeons, as well as ENT and head and neck specialists around the world will benefit from this work. Students and trainees will also benefit from studying this book cover to cover, while readers with advanced knowledge and experience will find it a useful reference.

My work with Dr. Yoshioka and other young surgeons from across the globe has been one of the most rewarding aspects of my career and a source of many treasured friendships. This book is a reflection of this friendship and cooperation.

Albert L. Rhoton, Jr., MD

Intracranial Region and Skull

1 Intracranial Region

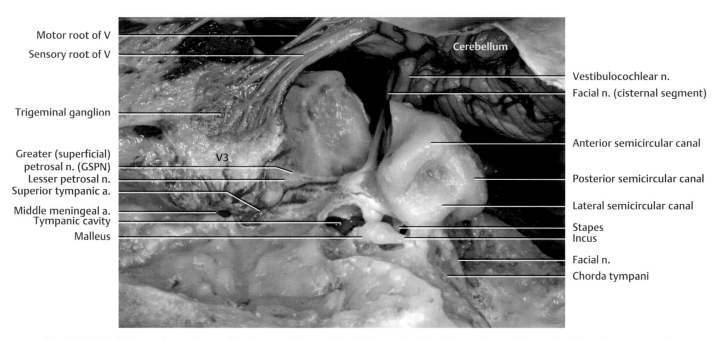

Motor root of V
Sensory root of V

Cerebellum

Vestibulocochlear n.
Facial n. (cisternal segment)

Trigeminal ganglion

Anterior semicircular canal

Greater (superficial)
petrosal n. (GSPN)
Lesser petrosal n.
Superior tympanic a.

V3

Posterior semicircular canal

Lateral semicircular canal

Middle meningeal a.
Tympanic cavity
Malleus

Stapes
Incus

Facial n.
Chorda tympani

Fig. 1.1. Middle fossa from above. The tegmen tympani and the roof of the internal acoustic meatus have been opened.

The facial nerve contains motor fibers, which are responsible for facial expression, as well as other nerve fibers involved in sensation (auricular concha; see **Fig. 13.3b**), taste (anterior two-thirds of the tongue; see **Fig. 1.3**), and secretory function (lacrimal gland, submandibular gland, and sublingual gland; see **Fig. 5.9a** and **Fig. 12.1**).

The facial nerve emerges from the brainstem at the junction of the pons and medulla. The course of the facial nerve may be divided into intracranial, intratemporal, and extratemporal segments. The intracranial segment, known as the pontine or cisternal segment, spans roughly 25 mm and connects the facial nerve from its origin to the entrance of the internal acoustic meatus. The intratemporal segment can be divided into four segments: meatal, labyrinthine, horizontal, and vertical. The facial nerve, accompanied by the vestibulocochlear nerve, enters the temporal bone through the internal acoustic meatus. Initially, there are two separate components, which are the motor root supplying the muscle of the face and the nervus intermedius that contains sensory fibers concerned with the perception of taste and parasympathetic (secretomotor) fibers to the lacrimal, submandibular, and

sublingual glands. The two components merge within the meatus.

The greater (superficial) petrosal nerve (GSPN) is a branch of the facial nerve and carries parasympathetic fibers to the pterygopalatine fossa. It emerges within the facial canal of the temporal bone, close to the geniculate ganglion of the facial nerve. It then passes through the bone to appear on the floor of the middle cranial fossa and runs medially in a shallow groove to the foramen lacerum. Passing within the foramen lacerum, the greater petrosal nerve enters the pterygoid canal that lies at the base of the pterygoid process. On leaving the pterygoid canal, the nerve emerges into the pterygopalatine fossa and joins the pterygopalatine ganglion (see **Fig. 10.15**).

The lesser petrosal nerve is a branch of the glossopharyngeal nerve and carries parasympathetic fibers to the otic ganglion. The nerve arises in the middle ear and passes on to the floor of the middle cranial fossa through a hiatus in the petrous part of the temporal bone. The nerve lies in a groove located lateral to that of the greater petrosal nerve and runs toward the foramen ovale and then enters the infratemporal fossa through the foramen ovale to join the otic ganglion (see **Fig. 10.12**).

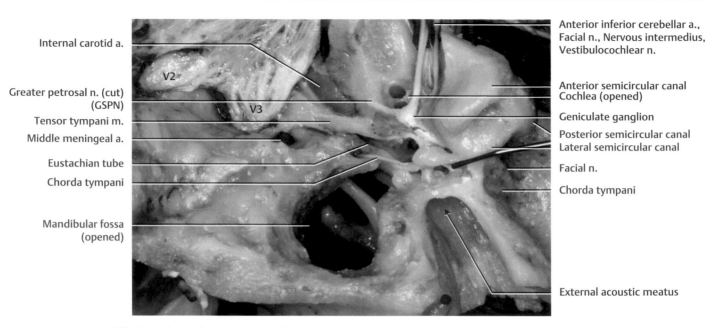

Internal carotid a.

V2

Greater petrosal n. (cut) (GSPN)

Tensor tympani m.

Middle meningeal a.

V3

Eustachian tube

Chorda tympani

Mandibular fossa (opened)

Anterior inferior cerebellar a., Facial n., Nervous intermedius, Vestibulocochlear n.

Anterior semicircular canal Cochlea (opened)

Geniculate ganglion

Posterior semicircular canal Lateral semicircular canal

Facial n.

Chorda tympani

External acoustic meatus

Fig. 1.2. Middle fossa from above. The mandibular fossa and the roof of external acoustic meatus have been opened.

The trigeminal nerve supplies sensations to the face, mucous membranes, and other structures of the head. It is the motor nerve for the muscles of mastication and contains proprioceptive fibers. It exits the brain by a large sensory root and a smaller motor root emerging from the pons at its junction with the middle cerebral peduncle. It passes laterally to join the trigeminal (gasserian or semilunar) ganglion in the trigeminal cave (Meckel's cave) close to the apex of the petrous part of the temporal bone, and then it appears as three major (ophthalmic, maxillary and mandibular) divisions. After removing the dura, the maxillary (V2) and mandibular (V3) nerves are identified. The ophthalmic and maxillary nerves pass through the lateral wall of the cavernous sinus. The mandibular nerve passes directly to the foramen ovale.

The tensor tympani muscle lies within a bony canal situated above the Eustachian tube in the anterior wall of the tympanic cavity. It draws the handle of the malleus medially, and the muscle tenses the tympanic membrane and helps to damp sound vibrations. The nerve to the tensor tympani muscle is derived from the mandibular division of the trigeminal nerve.

The middle meningeal artery, which is a branch of the maxillary artery (mandibular segment), enters the middle cranial fossa through the foramen spinosum. This artery has branches to the trigeminal ganglion and to the tympanic cavity (superior tympanic branch). The superior tympanic artery supplies the tensor tympani muscle. An accessory meningeal artery, which is a branch of the maxillary artery (mandibular segment), runs through the foramen ovale into the middle cranial fossa to supply the trigeminal ganglion and the dura lining the floor of the middle cranial fossa.

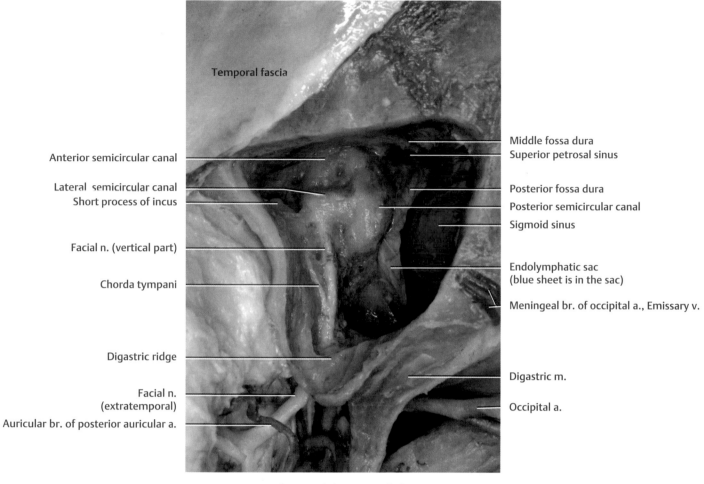

Anterior semicircular canal

Lateral semicircular canal
Short process of incus

Facial n. (vertical part)

Chorda tympani

Digastric ridge

Facial n.
(extratemporal)
Auricular br. of posterior auricular a.

Temporal fascia

Middle fossa dura
Superior petrosal sinus

Posterior fossa dura
Posterior semicircular canal
Sigmoid sinus

Endolymphatic sac
(blue sheet is in the sac)

Meningeal br. of occipital a., Emissary v.

Digastric m.

Occipital a.

Fig. 1.3. Lateral view of the mastoid after mastoidectomy

The mastoid process is a prominence projecting from the undersurface of the mastoid portion of the temporal bone. This process is a point of attachment for the splenius capitis, the longissimus capitis, the digastric posterior belly, and the sternocleidomastoid muscles.

The chorda tympani is given off just before the stylomastoid foramen. It is the branch from the nervus intermedius. It contains parasympathetic fibers going to the submandibular ganglion and taste fibers from the anterior two-thirds of the tongue. It initially runs within its own canal before entering the tympanic cavity to cross the malleus. It then enters another canal before leaving the temporal bone through the petrotympanic (squamotympanic) fissure.

Within the facial canal, close to the pyramid, arises the nerve to the stapedius muscle. The stapedius is the smallest skeletal muscle in the human body. At just over 1 mm in length, its purpose is to stabilize the smallest bone in the body, the stapes. This muscle helps to damp excessive sound vibrations and functions when sound is too loud.

The digastric ridge corresponds to the digastric groove and marks the location of the facial canal just anterior to it. This is a ridge of bone just deep or medial to the mastoid tip.

Hypoglossal-facial nerve side-to-end anastomosis without nerve grafting can be performed to cut the facial nerve at the point just below the lateral semicircular canal.

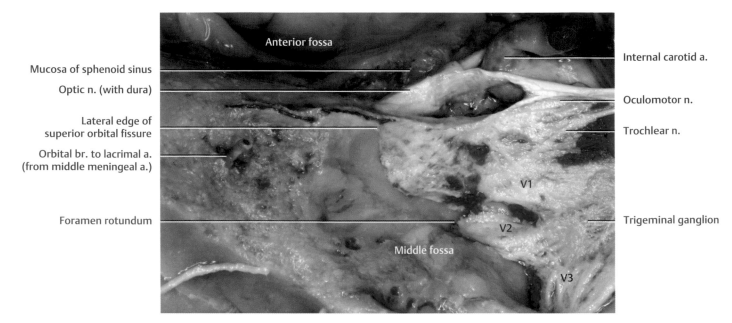

Mucosa of sphenoid sinus

Optic n. (with dura)

Lateral edge of
superior orbital fissure

Orbital br. to lacrimal a.
(from middle meningeal a.)

Foramen rotundum

Anterior fossa

Internal carotid a.

Oculomotor n.

Trochlear n.

V1

V2

Middle fossa

Trigeminal ganglion

V3

Fig. 1.4. The superior orbital fissure and trigeminal nerve. The optic canal has been opened, and anterior clinoidectomy has been done.

The trigeminal nerve has three divisions: ophthalmic (V1), maxillary (V2), and mandibular (V3). The ophthalmic nerve passes into the orbit through the superior orbital fissure. The maxillary nerve passes into the pterygopalatine fossa through the foramen rotundum. The mandibular nerve passes into the infratemporal fossa through the foramen ovale. All divisions have meningeal branches. The dura mater is innervated by the meningeal branches mainly from the trigeminal nerves.

The motor division of the mandibular nerve supplies the muscles of mastication: masseter, temporalis, pterygoid, mylohyoid, and digastric. These muscles produce elevation, depression, protrusion, retraction, and the side-to-side movements of the mandible. The motor division also supplies the tensor tympani and tensor veli palatini muscles.

The meningo-orbital foramen is located in the lateral wall of the orbit and links the orbit to the cranial cavity. It represents a passage for the artery connecting the orbital branch of the anterior division of the middle meningeal artery and lacrimal branch of the ophthalmic artery.

2 Skull: External and Internal Views

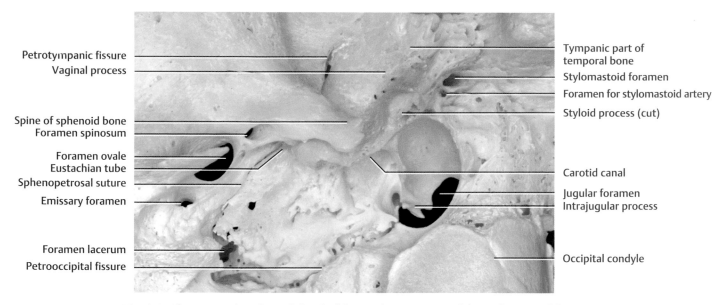

Petrotympanic fissure

Vaginal process

Spine of sphenoid bone
Foramen spinosum

Foramen ovale
Eustachian tube
Sphenopetrosal suture
Emissary foramen

Foramen lacerum
Petrooccipital fissure

Tympanic part of
temporal bone
Stylomastoid foramen
Foramen for stylomastoid artery
Styloid process (cut)

Carotid canal

Jugular foramen
Intrajugular process

Occipital condyle

Fig. 2.1. The external surface of the skull base. Close-up view of the stylomastoid foramen.

The facial nerve exits from the stylomastoid foramen and is supplied by the stylomastoid artery, which usually originates from the posterior auricular artery. The stylomastoid artery enters into the skull from the foramen adjacent to the stylomastoid foramen.

The foramen ovale allows passage between the middle cranial fossa and the infratemporal fossa of the mandibular division of the trigeminal nerve, the lesser petrosal branch of the glossopharyngeal nerve, the accessory meningeal branch of the maxillary artery, and some emissary veins. Behind the foramen ovale lies the foramen spinosum, which transmits the middle meningeal vessels and meningeal branch of the mandibular division of the trigeminal nerve.

The jugular foramen is located between the temporal bone and the occipital bone. The structures that traverse the jugular foramen are the sigmoid sinus and jugular bulb, the inferior petrosal sinus, the meningeal branches of the ascending pharyngeal and occipital arteries, the glossopharyngeal, vagus, and accessory nerves with their ganglia, the tympanic branch of the glossopharyngeal nerve (Jacobson's nerve), the auricular branch (also known as the mastoid branch) of the vagus nerve (Arnold's nerve), and the cochlear aqueduct. The intrajugular process is a small, curved process which partially or completely divides the jugular foramen into lateral and medial parts.

Behind the foramen spinosum, the bone is raised to form the spine of the sphenoid to which the sphenomandibular ligament is attached. The posterior margin here is grooved and is related to the cartilaginous component of the Eustachian tube (see **Fig. 10.18**).

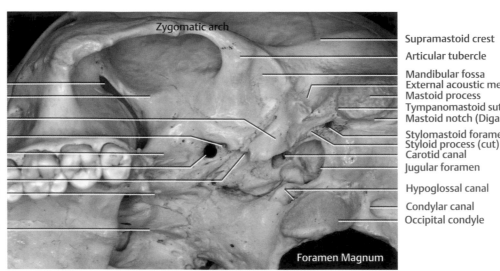

Zygomatic arch

Supramastoid crest
Articular tubercle

Inferior orbital fissure
Infratemporal crest
Vaginal process
(Tympanic part)
Foramen spinosum
Lateral pterygoid plate
Foramen ovale
Eustachian tube
Pterygoid hamulus

Mandibular fossa
External acoustic meatus
Mastoid process
Tympanomastoid suture (Drop-off point)
Mastoid notch (Digastric Groove)
Stylomastoid foramen
Styloid process (cut)
Carotid canal
Jugular foramen
Hypoglossal canal
Condylar canal
Occipital condyle

Vomer

Foramen Magnum

Fig. 2.2. Infratemporal fossa. The mandible has been removed.

The digastric muscle is attached to the mastoid notch (digastric groove), the anterior end of which indicates the stylomastoid foramen. The tympanomastoid suture is a landmark of facial nerve trunk. The facial nerve (stylomastoid foramen) can be identified at 6 to 8 mm medial to the inferior "drop-off" point of the tympanomastoid suture.

Jacobson's nerve arises from the petrous ganglion of the glossopharyngeal nerve. It enters the tympanic cavity via the inferior tympanic canaliculus and contributes to the tympanic plexus. It contains both sensory and parasympathetic fibers. The sensory fibers supply the middle ear. The parasympathetic fibers leave the plexus as the lesser petrosal nerve and enter the otic ganglion.

Arnold's nerve originates from the superior ganglion of the vagus nerve below the jugular foramen. It passes behind the internal jugular vein and ascends through the mastoid canaliculus on the lateral wall of the jugular fossa. It traverses the substance of the temporal bone and crosses the facial canal

above the stylomastoid foramen, where it gives off a branch that joins the facial nerve. The nerve finally reaches the surface by passing through the tympanomastoid suture. It divides into two branches: one joins the posterior auricular nerve, while the other innervates the skin of the concha and a small area of the cranial surface near the mastoid (see **Fig. 13.3**).

The osseous boundaries of the infratemporal fossa are the posterolateral maxillary surface anteriorly, the lateral pterygoid plate anteromedially, the mandibular ramus laterally, and the tympanic part of the temporal bone and the styloid process posteriorly. The fossa is domed anteriorly by the infratemporal surface of the greater sphenoid wing, the site of the foramina ovale and spinosum, and posteriorly by the squamous part of the temporal bone. The inferior, posteromedial, and superolateral aspects are open without bony walls. The infratemporal crest is the boundary between the temporal fossa and infratemporal fossa.

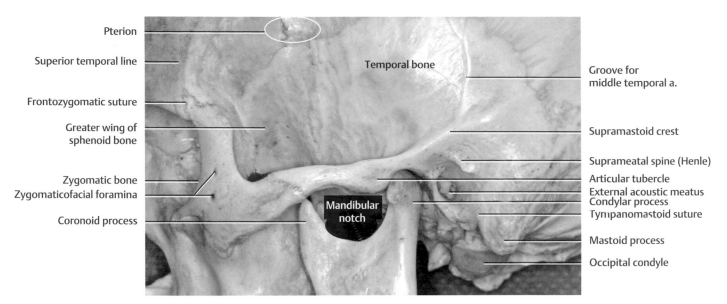

Pterion
Superior temporal line
Frontozygomatic suture
Greater wing of
sphenoid bone
Zygomatic bone
Zygomaticofacial foramina
Coronoid process

Temporal bone
Mandibular
notch

Groove for
middle temporal a.
Supramastoid crest
Suprameatal spine (Henle)
Articular tubercle
External acoustic meatus
Condylar process
Tympanomastoid suture
Mastoid process
Occipital condyle

Fig. 2.3. Lateral view of the skull with the temporal bone highlighted.

The suprameatal triangle, a depressed area located below the anterior part of the supramastoid crest and behind the posterosuperior margin of the external acoustic meatus, marks the deep location of the mastoid antrum. The suprameatal spine (the spine of Henle), which locates anterior part of the suprameatal triangle, approximates the deep site of the tympanic facial nerve segment and the lateral canal.

The zygomaticofacial nerve is a sensory nerve of the cheek and one of the two branches of the zygomatic nerve that originated from the maxillary nerve. It comes out to the face through the zygomaticofacial foramen. This foramen is sometimes doubled, and this figure shows two zygomaticofacial foramina.

Pterion is the landmark for frontotemporal craniotomy. It is the H-shaped region where the four calvarial bones (frontal, sphenoid, parietal, and temporal) meet.

The superior temporal line begins at the zygomatic process of the frontal bone and first curves superoposteriorly and then inferiorly and anteriorly to the supramastoid crest. It provides attachment for temporal fascia.

The groove for the middle temporal artery, which supplies posterior and upper part of temporalis muscle, is sometimes prominent on the temporal bone.

The base of the temporomandibular ligament is attached to the zygomatic process of the temporal bone and the articular tubercle (see **Fig. 9.1**).

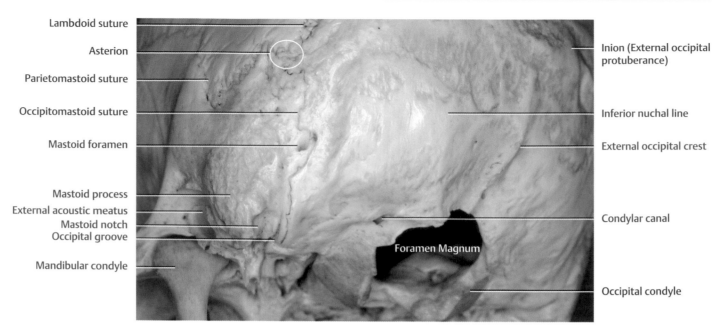

Lambdoid suture

Asterion

Parietomastoid suture

Occipitomastoid suture

Mastoid foramen

Mastoid process

External acoustic meatus

Mastoid notch

Occipital groove

Mandibular condyle

Inion (External occipital protuberance)

Inferior nuchal line

External occipital crest

Foramen Magnum

Condylar canal

Occipital condyle

Fig. 2.4. Posterolateral view of the skull.

The mastoid notch (digastric groove), where the digastric muscle is attached, and the occipital groove, where the occipital artery courses on, are parallel grooves on the posterior aspect of the mastoid process.

The meningeal branch of the occipital artery and emissary vein penetrate the cranium through the mastoid foramen.

The asterion located at the junction of the lambdoid, occipitomastoid, and parietomastoid sutures is usually located over the junction of the lower part of the transverse and sigmoid sinuses.

The external occipital protuberance is a projection of the external surface of the occipital squama. It is situated approximately at the mid-point of the squama. It provides attachment for the medial fibers of the trapezius muscle. Below this prominence is a crest that runs inferiorly to the back edge of the foramen magnum. This crest, called the external occipital crest, provides attachment for the nuchal ligament.

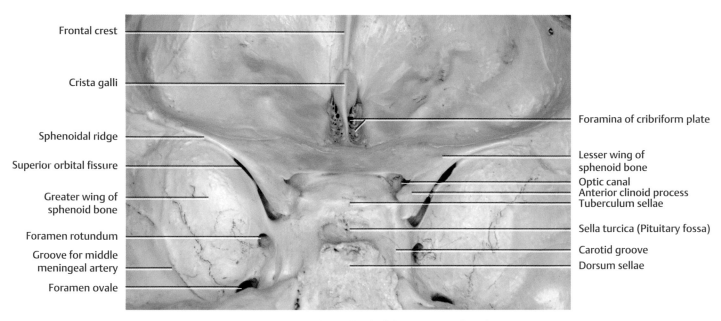

Frontal crest

Crista galli

Sphenoidal ridge

Superior orbital fissure

Greater wing of sphenoid bone

Foramen rotundum

Groove for middle meningeal artery

Foramen ovale

Foramina of cribriform plate

Lesser wing of sphenoid bone

Optic canal
Anterior clinoid process
Tuberculum sellae

Sella turcica (Pituitary fossa)

Carotid groove
Dorsum sellae

Fig. 2.5. Anterior and middle skull base (internal surface).

The sensory innervation of the face is via the three divisions of the trigeminal nerve: ophthalmic, maxillary, and mandibular.

The superior orbital fissure lies between the greater and lesser wings of the sphenoid at the junction of the roof and lateral wall of the orbit. It transmits the oculomotor nerve, the trochlear nerve, and the sympathetic filaments from the internal carotid plexus, the abducens nerve, and the ophthalmic division of the trigeminal nerve, together with the ophthalmic veins. It may also transmit the orbital branch of the middle meningeal artery and the recurrent branch of the lacrimal artery (see **Fig. 3.1**).

The foramen rotundum lies within the greater wing of the sphenoid. It allows communication between the middle cranial fossa and the pterygopalatine fossa. The maxillary division of the trigeminal nerve passes through the foramen.

The foramen ovale is also in the greater wing of the sphenoid, and it communicates between the middle cranial fossa above and the infratemporal fossa below. The mandibular division of the trigeminal nerve, the lesser petrosal branch of the glossopharyngeal nerve, the accessory meningeal branch

of the maxillary artery, and an emissary vein from the cavernous sinus to the pterygoid venous plexus pass through the foramen.

The ophthalmic nerve supplies the forehead, upper eyelid, and dorsum of the nose. The maxillary nerve supplies the lower eyelid, the cheek, the upper lip, the ala of the nose, and part of the temple, the maxillary teeth, and the nasal cavity. The mandibular nerve has motor and sensory fibers. The latter supplies the skin over the mandible, the lower cheek, part of the temple and ear, the lower teeth, the gingival mucosa, and the lower lip.

The crista galli is the thick crest of bone that projects above the cribriform. The crest is thickest near its base and tapers superiorly. It projects between the two cerebral hemispheres with the falx cerebri attaching to its posterior margin.

The frontal crest is an anterior crest of bone in the midline of the internal surface of the frontal bone. This sharp ridge of bone is a continuation of the converging edges of the sulcus for the superior sagittal sinus. The anterior part of the falx cerebri attaches to the ridge.

3 Orbit and Facial Bone

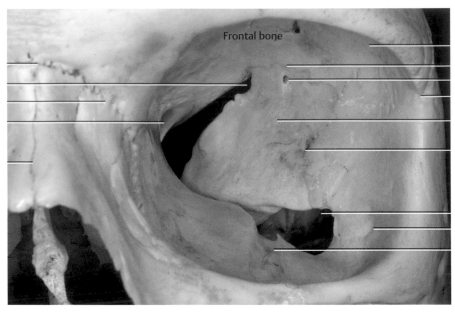

Frontal bone

Frontonasal suture
Superior orbital fissure
Frontomaxillary suture
Optic canal
Internasal suture

Fossa for lacrimal gland
Sphenofrontal suture
Meningo-orbital foramen
Frontozygomatic suture
Greater wing of sphenoid bone
Sphenozygomatic suture

Inferior orbital fissure
Zygomatico-orbital foramen
Infraorbital sulcus (groove)

Fig. 3.1. Anterior view of the orbit.

The inferior orbital fissure lies at the junction of the lateral wall and the floor of the orbit. Through this fissure pass the infraorbital and zygomatic branches of the maxillary division of the trigeminal nerve and accompanying vessels.

The infraorbital nerve is the terminal branch of the maxillary nerve. It courses along the orbital floor in the infraorbital sulcus (groove) into a canal and onto the face at the infraorbital foramen.

The zygomatic nerve arises from the maxillary nerve in the pterygopalatine fossa and passes through the inferior orbital fissure to course along the lateral wall of the orbit, where it divides into zygomaticofacial and zygomaticotemporal branches. The branches enter the zygomatico-orbital

foramina on the orbital surface of the zygomatic bone. When one foramen is present, the zygomatic vessels and nerve enter and then branch within the bone to exit different foramina as the zygomaticofacial and zygomaticotemporal vessels and nerve. The zygomaticotemporal nerve provides sensation to the temporal skin, and the zygomaticofacial nerve provides sensation to the skin over the prominence of the cheek.

Meningo-orbital foramen (lacrimal foramen) is located in the greater wing of the sphenoid, anterior to the tip of the superior orbital fissure, and is the source of an anastomosis between the lacrimal artery and the orbital branch of the middle meningeal artery. This foramen is present in approximately 50% of Caucasian people.

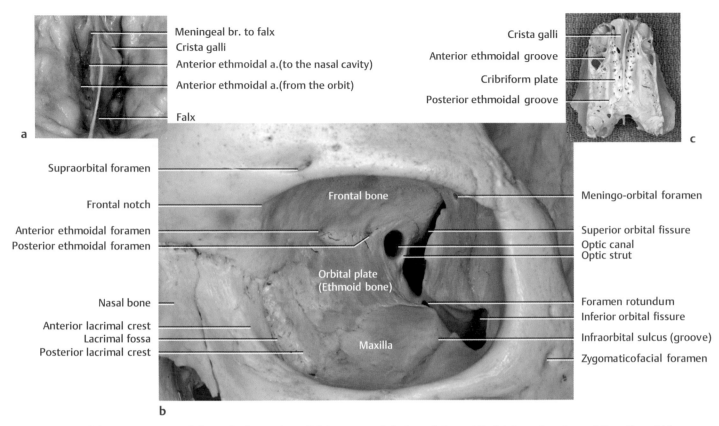

Fig. 3.2a-c. (a) Superior view of the cribriform plate. (b) Anteromedial view of the orbit. (c) Superior view of the ethmoid bone.

The supraorbital foramen, the frequency of which is 20 to 30%, is the passage mainly for the supraorbital nerve, especially its lateral branch, one of the medial branches, and its concomitant small artery (see **Fig. 5.3b**). The main trunk of the supraorbital artery generally passes under the supraorbital notch or just below the supraorbital rim. The supraorbital notch also transmits the supraorbital nerve. The frontal notch, which is medial to the supraorbital notch, transmits the supratrochlear nerve and artery.

The optic canal lies within the lesser wing of the sphenoid and transmits the optic nerve and ophthalmic artery.

The anterior and posterior ethmoidal foramina for the same nerves and vessels are situated at the medial wall. The anterior ethmoidal nerve exits the orbit through the anterior ethmoidal foramen and enters the anterior cranial fossa. It runs into the roof of the nose through small slits lying on each side of the crista galli. The posterior ethmoidal nerve exits the orbit

through the posterior ethmoidal foramen to enter the nose. It supplies the sphenoidal sinus and the posterior ethmoidal air cells. The view of the ethmoid bone from above (**Fig. 3.2c**) shows anterior and posterior ethmoidal grooves for the same nerves and vessels, which are converted into foramina by articulation with frontal bone. It is important that lowest point of the cribriform plate (lowest point of the anterior skull base) is generally below the anterior and posterior ethmoidal foramen on the medial orbital wall (**Fig. 3.2a**).

The fossa for the lacrimal sac is formed by the lacrimal incisure on the maxilla and a matching groove on the lacrimal bone. When the adjacent grooves are combined, they form a fossa and a canal that houses the lacrimal sac and transmits the beginning of the lacrimal duct toward the nasal cavity.

The cribriform plate is the horizontal plate of the ethmoid bone perforated with numerous foramina for the passage of the olfactory nerve filaments from the nasal cavity.

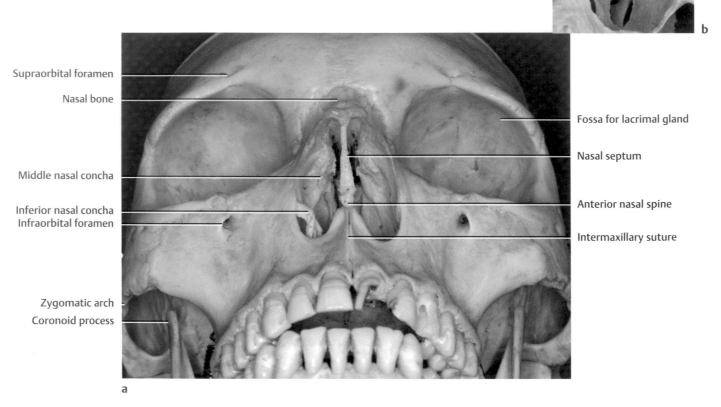

Supraorbital foramen

Nasal bone

Fossa for lacrimal gland

Nasal septum

Middle nasal concha

Inferior nasal concha
Infraorbital foramen

Anterior nasal spine

Intermaxillary suture

Zygomatic arch
Coronoid process

a

b

Fig. 3.3a,b. (a) Anteroinferior view of the skull. **(b)** Anteroinferior view of the maxilla after removing the anterior and posterior sinus walls to show the foramen rotundum.

The infraorbital foramen lies below the infraorbital rim. The infraorbital branch of the maxillary nerve and infraorbital vessels pass through the foramen.

The anterior and posterior walls of the left maxillary sinus have been opened to see the pterygopalatine fossa and foramen rotundum (**Fig. 3.3b**). Black string is passing from the foramen rotundum to the infraorbital foramen. The pterygopalatine fossa is a cone-shaped paired depression deep to the infratemporal fossa and posterior to the maxilla on each side of the skull, located between the pterygoid process and the maxillary tuberosity, close to the apex of the orbit. It is the indented area medial to the pterygomaxillary fissure leading into the sphenopalatine foramen. It communicates with the nasal and oral cavities, the infratemporal fossa, the orbit, the pharynx, and the middle cranial fossa through eight foramina (see **Fig. 8.4**).

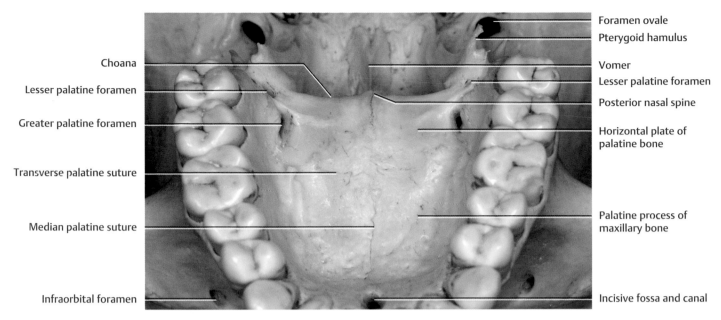

Choana
Lesser palatine foramen
Greater palatine foramen
Transverse palatine suture
Median palatine suture
Infraorbital foramen

Foramen ovale
Pterygoid hamulus
Vomer
Lesser palatine foramen
Posterior nasal spine
Horizontal plate of palatine bone
Palatine process of maxillary bone
Incisive fossa and canal

Fig. 3.4. Inferior view of the palatine bone.

The nasopalatine nerve, which is a branch of the pterygopalatine ganglion, enters the nasal cavity through the sphenopalatine foramen and runs obliquely downward and forward on the nasal septum. It terminates as the incisive nerve, which passes through the incisive canal with an accompany artery onto the hard palate to supply oral mucosa around the incisive papilla. It communicates with the corresponding nerve of the opposite side and with the greater palatine nerve.

The greater palatine nerve is a branch of the pterygopalatine ganglion that carries both general sensory and parasympathetic fibers. It passes through the grater palatine canal and onto the hard palate at the greater palatine foramen. It passes forward in a groove in the hard palate, nearly as far as the incisor teeth. It supplies the gums, the mucous membrane, and the glands of the hard palate, and it communicates in front with the terminal filaments of the nasopalatine nerve.

The lesser palatine nerve passes through the greater palatine canal and onto the palate at the lesser palatine foramen. It runs backward to supply the soft palate. It also has nasal branches that innervate the nasal cavity.

The pterygoid hamulus is the laterally deflected hook of bone at the inferior end of the medial pterygoid plate. It serves a pulley-like function for the tendon of the tensor veli palatini muscle and serves as the attachment for the pterygomandibular raphe.

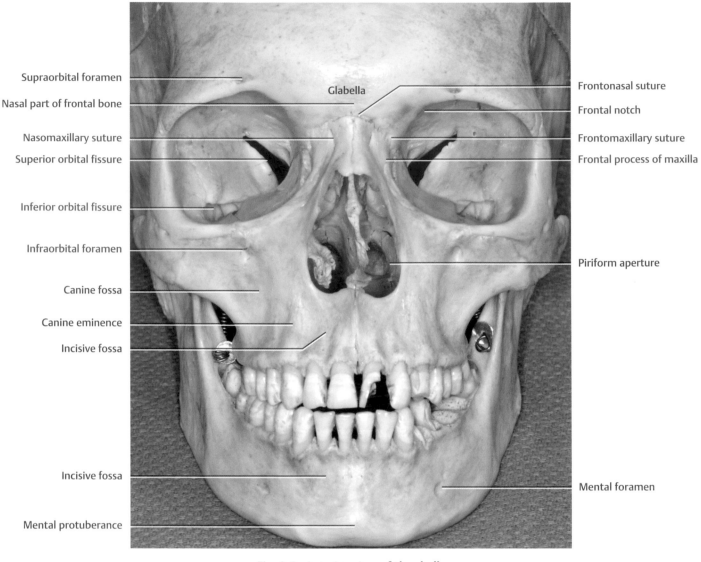

Supraorbital foramen

Nasal part of frontal bone

Nasomaxillary suture

Superior orbital fissure

Inferior orbital fissure

Infraorbital foramen

Canine fossa

Canine eminence

Incisive fossa

Incisive fossa

Mental protuberance

Glabella

Frontonasal suture

Frontal notch

Frontomaxillary suture

Frontal process of maxilla

Piriform aperture

Mental foramen

Fig. 3.5. Anterior view of the skull.

The orbicularis oculi muscle arises from the nasal part of the frontal bone, the frontal process of the maxilla, and the medial palpebral ligament.

The corrugator supercilii muscle arises from the medial end of the supraorbital ridge on the frontal bone.

The procerus muscle arises from the nasal bone and the lateral nasal cartilage.

The nasalis and depressor septi muscle arise from the maxilla in the region overlying the root of the lateral incisor and canine tooth.

The levator labii superioris muscle arises from the maxilla at the inferior orbital rim, above the infraorbital foramen.

The levator labii superioris alaeque nasi muscle arises from the frontal process of the maxilla.

The zygomaticus major muscle arises from the lateral surface of the zygomatic bone, just in front of the zygomaticotemporal suture. The zygomaticus minor muscle also arises from the zygomatic bone, just in front of the origin of zygomaticus major.

The canine eminence overlies the root of the canine tooth. It separates the anterior surface of the maxilla into two concave areas: a shallow, incisive fossa in front and a deeper, canine fossa behind. The levator anguli oris muscle arises from the canine fossa of the maxilla, immediately below the infraorbital foramen.

The supraorbital foramen, the infraorbital foramen, and the mental foramen are found approximately in line vertically.

The piriform aperture (anterior nasal aperture) is a heart- or pear-shaped bony nasal opening in the skull.

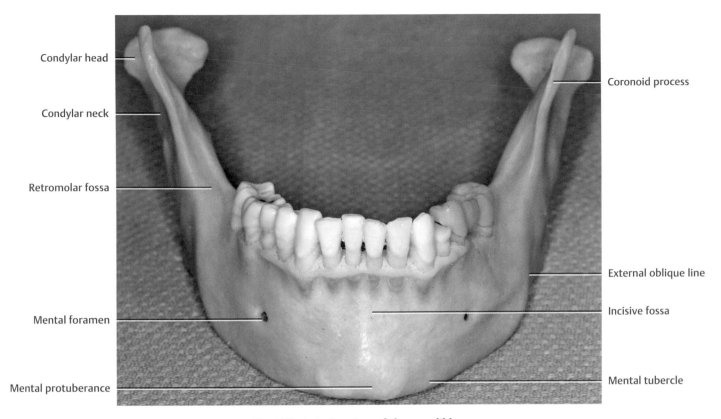

Condylar head

Condylar neck

Retromolar fossa

Mental foramen

Mental protuberance

Coronoid process

External oblique line

Incisive fossa

Mental tubercle

Fig. 3.6. Anterior view of the mandible.

The depressor labii inferioris muscle arises from the mandible just in front of the mental foramen.

The depressor anguli oris muscle arises from an extensive area around the external oblique line of the mandible.

The platysma muscle arises from the superficial fascia of the upper part of the thorax. It runs up to the neck to insert into the lower border of the body of the mandible, the skin of the lower part of the mouth, and the mimetic muscles around the angle of the mouth.

The mentalis muscle originates from the incisive fossa of the mandible.

The buccinator muscle is attached to the alveolar margin of the maxilla and mandible in the region of the molar teeth.

There are fibers by which the orbicularis oris muscle is connected with the maxilla and the septum of the nose above and with the mandible below.

A distinct prominence, the mental protuberance, lies at the inferior margin in the midline of the mandible. On each side of the protuberance are the mental tubercles. Above the mental protuberance lie a shallow depression called the incisive fossa. The mental foramen is in the region of the premolar teeth. The mental nerve, which originated from the inferior alveolar nerve, and the accompanying vessels pass onto the face through this foramen.

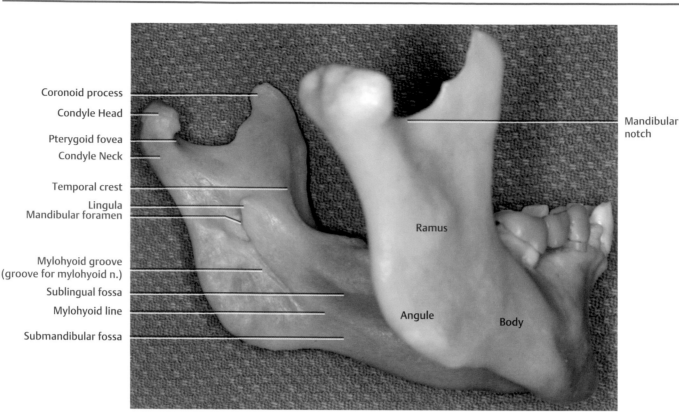

Coronoid process
Condyle Head
Pterygoid fovea
Condyle Neck
Temporal crest
Lingula
Mandibular foramen
Mylohyoid groove
(groove for mylohyoid n.)
Sublingual fossa
Mylohyoid line
Submandibular fossa

Mandibular notch

Ramus

Angle   Body

Fig. 3.7. Posterolateral view of the mandible.

The temporalis muscle inserts onto the apex, the anterior and posterior borders, and the medial surface of the coronoid process. The insertion extends down the anterior border of the ramus near the third molar tooth. Many of the fibers have a tendinous insertion. The temporal crest is a ridge along anteromedial aspect of the coronoid process and upper ramus of the mandible into which the temporalis muscle inserts.

A small depression, the pterygoid fovea, is a site of attachment of the lower head of lateral pterygoid muscle. It is situated on the anterior part of the neck of the condyle. The upper head of the lateral pterygoid muscle insets into the capsule and medial aspect of the articular disc of the temporomandibular joint.

The masseter muscle inserts into the lateral surface of the angle, ramus, and coronoid process of the mandible.

The medial pterygoid muscle inserts into the roughened surface of the angle of the mandible on its medial aspect.

The mandibular foramen, through which the inferior alveolar nerve and vessels pass into the mandibular canal, lies in the center of the medial surface of the ramus.

A bony process, the lingula, extends from the anterosuperior surface of the foramen and gives attachment to the sphenomandibular ligament.

The mylohyoid groove is where the mylohyoid nerve runs down from the posteroinferior surface of the mandibular foramen.

The sublingual gland lies adjacent to the sublingual fossa. The submandibular fossa is a depression for the submandibular gland.

II Upper Facial and Midfacial Region

4 Upper Facial and Midfacial Region Overview

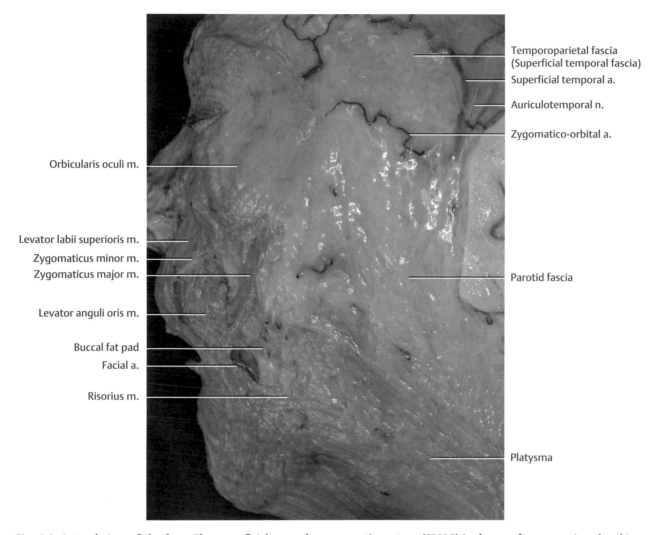

Temporoparietal fascia (Superficial temporal fascia)

Superficial temporal a.

Auriculotemporal n.

Zygomatico-orbital a.

Orbicularis oculi m.

Levator labii superioris m.

Zygomaticus minor m.

Zygomaticus major m.

Levator anguli oris m.

Buccal fat pad

Facial a.

Risorius m.

Parotid fascia

Platysma

Fig. 4.1. Lateral view of the face. The superficial musculoaponeurotic system (SMAS) is shown after removing the skin.

In the scalp, the superficial musculoaponeurotic system (SMAS) is represented by the galea aponeurotica, which then splits to ensheath the frontalis, the occipitalis, the procerus, and some of the periauricular muscles. In the temporal region, the SMAS, the superficial temporal fascia, and the temporoparietal fascia are synonymous. In the cheek, the SMAS is represented by the parotid fascia as a remnant of the primitive platysma. The SMAS is relatively thick over the parotid gland. However, it thins considerably, thereby making it difficult to dissect medially. The SMAS is continuous with the platysma below and extends to the zygoma above. The precise anatomy of the SMAS, its regional variations, and even the existence of the SMAS are still debated.

The facial nerve and its branches are under the SMAS. The frequency of appearance of certain mimetic muscle is known to vary. Some mimetic muscles, such as the levator labii superioris and the zygomaticus major, are almost always present, whereas the risorius muscle is relatively uncommon. Moreover, there is a striking degree of variability in their size and shape from individual to individual. Many of the mimetic muscles are attached to the facial skeleton and insert into the skin. Mimetic muscles cause movement of the facial skin to reflect emotions.

The risorius muscle does not arise from bone but originates from the connective tissue overlying the parotid gland. The muscle runs horizontally across the face to insert into the skin at the corner of the mouth. It pulls the corner of the mouth laterally, as in grinning.

The facial artery runs superficially above the SMAS layer at the buccal (on the buccinator muscle) and nasolabial (on the orbicularis oris muscle) region.

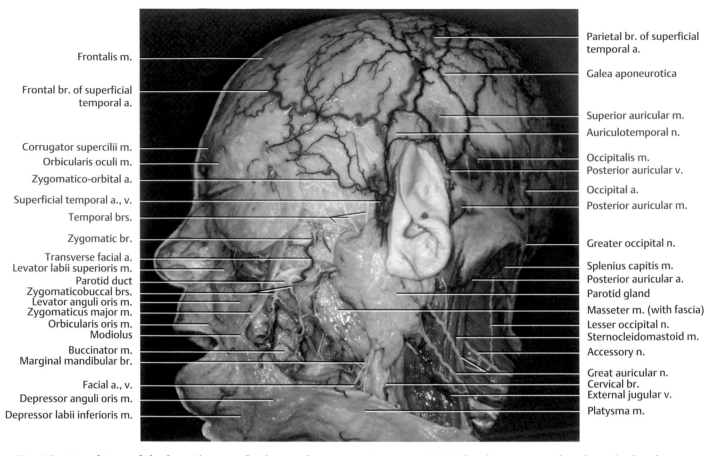

Frontalis m.

Frontal br. of superficial
temporal a.

Corrugator supercilii m.
Orbicularis oculi m.
Zygomatico-orbital a.
Superficial temporal a., v.
Temporal brs.
Zygomatic br.
Transverse facial a.
Levator labii superioris m.
Parotid duct
Zygomaticobuccal brs.
Levator anguli oris m.
Zygomaticus major m.
Orbicularis oris m.
Modiolus
Buccinator m.
Marginal mandibular br.
Facial a., v.
Depressor anguli oris m.
Depressor labii inferioris m.

Parietal br. of superficial
temporal a.

Galea aponeurotica

Superior auricular m.
Auriculotemporal n.

Occipitalis m.
Posterior auricular v.

Occipital a.
Posterior auricular m.

Greater occipital n.

Splenius capitis m.
Posterior auricular a.
Parotid gland
Masseter m. (with fascia)
Lesser occipital n.
Sternocleidomastoid m.
Accessory n.

Great auricular n.
Cervical br.
External jugular v.
Platysma m.

Fig. 4.2. Lateral view of the face. The superficial musculoaponeurotic system (SMAS) has been removed to show the facial nerve branches. Every mimetic muscle and part of the temporoparietal fascia and galea are preserved.

Mimetic muscles, with the exception of the buccinator, the levator anguli oris, and the mentalis, are innervated from their deep surface by the facial nerve branches. These muscles are located in the deepest layer among the mimic muscles and are innervated from their superficial surface. The superior auricular muscle arises from the temporoparietal fascia and inserts into the upper part of the cranial surface of the auricle. It is innervated by the temporal branch of the facial nerve. It displaces the auricle superiorly.

The facial artery and vein are independently running obliquely from the mandibular angle toward the medial canthus. The superficial temporal artery is one of the terminal branches of the external carotid artery. The artery passes upward toward the scalp, crossing the zygomatic process of the temporal bone. It divides into anterior (frontal) and posterior (parietal) branches. A transverse facial artery arises from the superficial artery within the parotid gland and crosses the masseter muscle above the parotid duct.

The superficial temporal vein is formed above the zygomatic arch by the union of anterior and posterior tributaries. The superficial temporal vein then enters the substance of the parotid gland. It unites first with the middle temporal vein and then with the maxillary vein to form the retromandibular vein in the gland. When the superficial temporal vein is poorly developed or, as occasionally happens, is absent, the posterior auricular vein usually compensates for it, as shown in this figure.

5 Forehead and Orbital Region

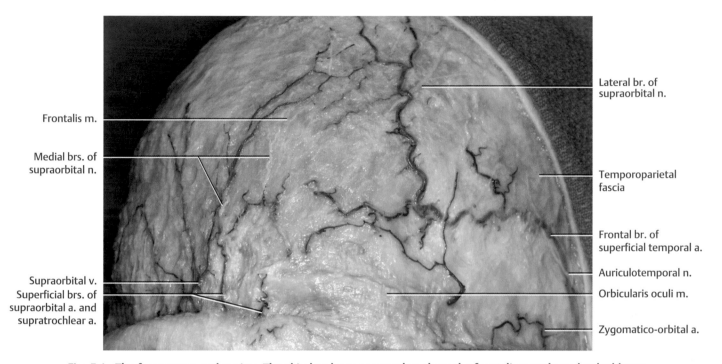

Frontalis m.

Medial brs. of
supraorbital n.

Supraorbital v.
Superficial brs. of
supraorbital a. and
supratrochlear a.

Lateral br. of
supraorbital n.

Temporoparietal
fascia

Frontal br. of
superficial temporal a.

Auriculotemporal n.

Orbicularis oculi m.

Zygomatico-orbital a.

Fig. 5.1. The frontotemporal region. The skin has been removed to show the frontalis muscle and galeal layer.

The galea aponeurotica extends from the external occipital protuberance and supreme nuchal lines to the eyebrows. The aponeurotica is continuous laterally with the temporoparietal fascia overlying the temporal fascia. The galea aponeurotica contains the occipitofrontal muscle. Each frontal belly of the frontalis muscle arises from the anterior margin of the galea aponeurotica and passes forward to merge with the orbicularis oculi muscle. The main function of the occipitofrontalis muscle is to elevate the eyebrows to produce transverse furrows of the forehead. This frontalis muscle is innervated by the temporal branch of the facial nerve.

The forehead sensation is supplied by the supraorbital and supratrochlear nerves. The supratrochlear nerve provides sensation to the medial side of the forehead. The supraorbital nerve has medial (superficial) and lateral (deep) branches. The former provides sensation to the forehead region, and the latter supplies sensation to the frontoparietal region. The lateral branch penetrates the frontalis muscle and galeal layer at the forehead, usually above the hairline.

The superficial temporal artery and vein run on the galeal aponeurotica. The superficial branches of the supraorbital and supratrochlear arteries communicate with the superficial temporal artery on the galeal layer.

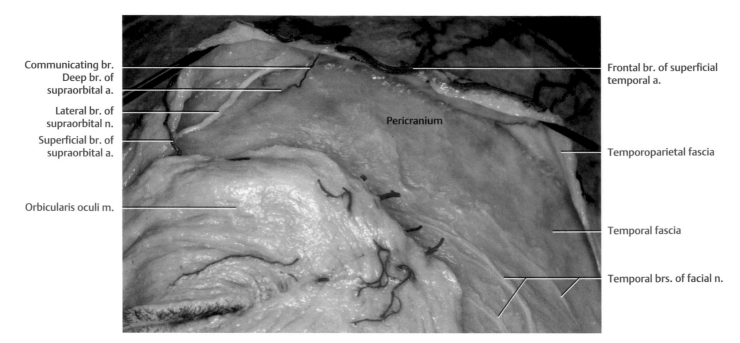

Communicating br.
Deep br. of supraorbital a.

Lateral br. of supraorbital n.

Superficial br. of supraorbital a.

Orbicularis oculi m.

Pericranium

Frontal br. of superficial temporal a.

Temporoparietal fascia

Temporal fascia

Temporal brs. of facial n.

Fig. 5.2. The frontotemporal region. The frontalis muscle has been separated from the orbicularis oculi muscle and lifted.

The temporal branches of the facial nerve generally course along the undersurface of the temporoparietal fascia and in the subgaleal fat pad. The temporoparietal fascia (galea) and its extension frontalis muscle are elevated to leave the temporal branches of the facial nerve on the temporal fascia in this specimen.

The deep (lateral) division of the supraorbital nerve runs cephalad across the lateral forehead between the frontalis muscle and galeal layer and the pericranium as the sensory nerve to the frontoparietal scalp. There is a loose areolar tissue between the galea aponeurotica and the pericranium that allows scalp mobility.

The arterial communication between the superficial temporal artery and the deep branch of the supraorbital artery is shown.

The pericranium is continuous with the temporal fascia in the temporal region.

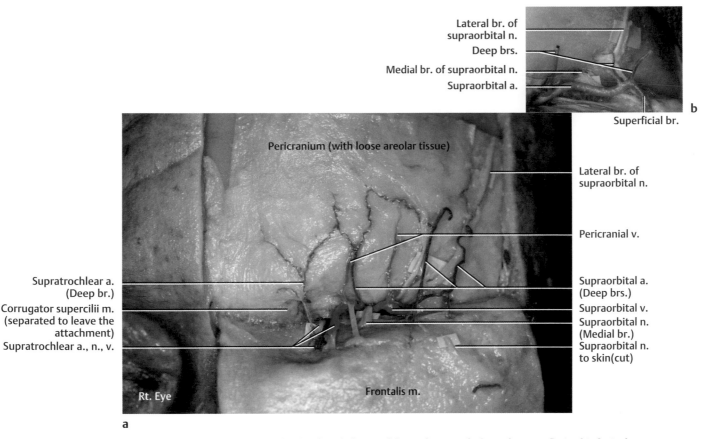

Fig. 5.3a,b. **(a) The supraorbital region. The forehead skin and frontalis muscle have been reflected inferiorly. (b) Medial view of the supraorbital region.**

The frontalis muscle has been reflected inferiorly. The attachment of the corrugator supercilii muscle is shown at the medial side on the frontal bone.

The supraorbital nerve has two divisions: a superficial (medial) division that passes shortly over the pericranium and then pierces the frontalis muscle, providing sensory supply to the forehead skin, and a deep (lateral) division that runs cephalad across the lateral forehead between the galea aponeurotica and the pericranium as the sensory nerve to the frontoparietal scalp. The deep division consistently courses approximately 1 cm medial to the superior temporal line, which is the attachment of the temporal fascia. It can be identified at the level of hair line just beneath the galea aponeurotica. In contrast, the supratrochlear nerve has only a superficial branch.

The main trunk of the supraorbital and supratrochlear arteries course below the orbital roof and divide near or above the supraorbital rim into superficial and deep branches (**Fig. 5.3b**). The superficial branch run in the galea-frontalis layer of the scalp, and the deep branches ascend in and supply the pericranium. The deep branch of the supratrochlear artery generally penetrates the corrugator supercilii muscle before reaching the pericranium. The forehead pericranium is supplied dominantly from the deep branches of the supraorbital artery.

Both the deep veins from the pericranial layer and the superficial veins from the galea-frontalis layer empty into a transverse channel in the supraorbital area that courses between the galea-frontalis layer and the pericranium. This transverse venous trunk joins the supratrochlear veins on the medial side and the superficial temporal veins on the lateral side.

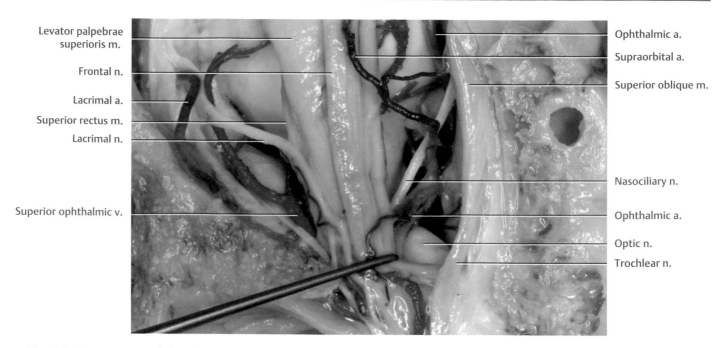

Levator palpebrae superioris m.

Frontal n.

Lacrimal a.

Superior rectus m.

Lacrimal n.

Superior ophthalmic v.

Ophthalmic a.

Supraorbital a.

Superior oblique m.

Nasociliary n.

Ophthalmic a.

Optic n.

Trochlear n.

Fig. 5.4. Superior view of the orbit without orbital fat. Extraocular muscles above the optic nerve have been retracted laterally to show the ophthalmic artery.

The ophthalmic nerve passes along the lateral dural wall of the cavernous sinus and gives off three main branches just before the superior orbital fissure. The three branches are the lacrimal nerve, the frontal nerve, and the nasociliary nerve.

The lacrimal nerve enters the orbit through the superior orbital fissure. It passes forward along the lateral wall of the orbit on the superior border of the lateral rectus muscle. It passes through the lacrimal gland to supply the conjunctiva and the skin of the lateral part of the upper eyelid. The lacrimal nerve communicates with the zygomaticotemporal branch of the maxillary nerve. The parasympathetic fivers to the lacrimal gland are conveyed via the zygomatic branch of the maxillary nerve.

The frontal nerve enters the orbit through the superior orbital fissure and passes forward on the levator palpebrae superioris muscle. It divides into the supraorbital and the supratrochlear nerves.

The nasociliary nerve passes into the orbit through the superior orbital fissure and runs forward and medially across the optic nerve. The nasociliary nerve gives rise to the sensory branches to the ciliary ganglion, the long ciliary branches, and the posterior ethmoidal nerves. The posterior ethmoidal nerve leaves the orbit through the posterior ethmoidal foramen to enter the nose. It supplies the sphenoidal sinus and the posterior ethmoidal air cells. Near the anterior ethmoidal foramen, the nasociliary nerve divides into its terminal branches: the anterior ethmoidal and the infratrochlear nerves.

The ophthalmic artery arises from the internal carotid artery, and it traverses the optic canal below the optic nerve. It passes from the lateral side to the medial side immediately beneath the superior rectus muscle. Then, it runs with the nasociliary nerve and passes between the superior oblique and medial rectus muscles. The ophthalmic artery terminates near the medial canthus by dividing into the dorsal nasal and the supratrochlear arteries.

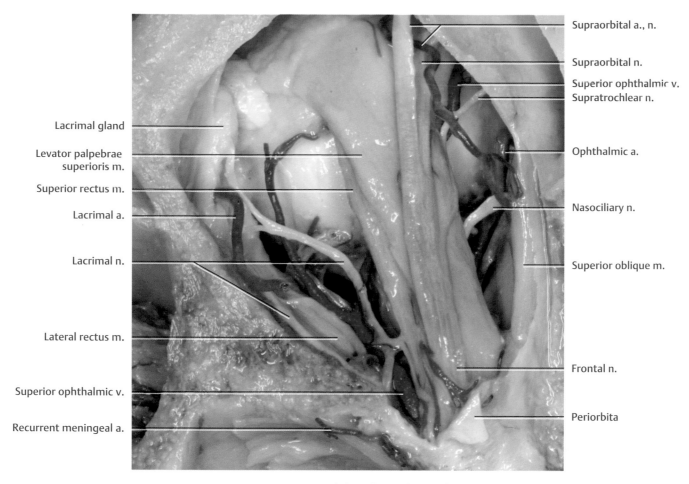

Labels on image:
Supraorbital a., n.
Supraorbital n.
Superior ophthalmic v.
Supratrochlear n.
Ophthalmic a.
Nasociliary n.
Superior oblique m.
Frontal n.
Periorbita
Lacrimal gland
Levator palpebrae superioris m.
Superior rectus m.
Lacrimal a.
Lacrimal n.
Lateral rectus m.
Superior ophthalmic v.
Recurrent meningeal a.

Fig. 5.5. Superior view of the orbit without orbital fat.

The supraorbital nerve emerges from the orbit through the supraorbital notch and foramen (only some of its branches always pass through whenever there is a foramen [see **Fig. 5.3**]). It supplies most of the forehead and upper lid, except for its lateral region.

The supratrochlear nerve emerges from the orbit above the trochlea and gives a descending branch to the infratrochlear nerve. It ascends onto the medial part of the forehead through the frontal notch.

The nasociliary nerve divides into the anterior ethmoidal and the infratrochlear nerves near the anterior ethmoidal foramen.

The infratrochlear nerve passes forward along the medial wall of the orbit below the pulley of the superior oblique muscle. It passes above the medial palpebral ligament to reach the side of the nose to supply the skin of the medial aspect of the upper eyelid.

The anterior ethmoidal nerve exits the orbit through the anterior ethmoidal foramen. It enters the anterior cranial fossa where the cribriform plate of the ethmoid bone meets the orbital part of the frontal bone. It then runs into the roof of the nose through a small foramen at the side of the crista galli. The anterior ethmoidal nerve terminates on the face as the external nasal nerve to supply the skin of the nasal tip.

The ophthalmic artery gives rise to four branches within the orbit to supply the face: the lacrimal artery, the supraorbital artery, the supratrochlear artery, and the dorsal nasal artery. The lacrimal artery reaches the skin through the upper lateral corner of the orbit and supplies the lateral part of the eyelids. Within the orbit, the lacrimal artery gives off zygomaticofacial and zygomaticotemporal arteries.

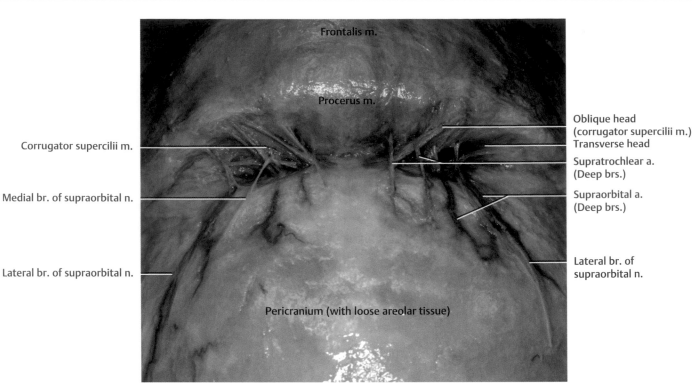

Fig. 5.6. The supraorbital region. The skin and frontalis muscle have been reflected.

The corrugator supercilii muscle originates from the medial end of the supraorbital ridge on the frontal bone, deep to the orbicularis oculi muscle. It passes upward and outward through the orbicularis oculi muscle to insert into the skin of the middle of the eyebrow. This muscle has two muscle bellies: a transverse head and an oblique head. This muscle produces vertical ridges above the bridge of the nose when frowning by drawing the eyebrow downward and inward.

The frontalis muscle mingles with the corrugator supercilii and orbicularis oculi muscles. The medial fibers of frontalis muscle are continuous with procerus muscle.

The lateral branch of the supraorbital nerve, which supplies the frontoparietal scalp, courses obliquely along the superior temporal line on the pericranium with concomitant artery. The lateral division consistently courses approximately 1 cm medial to the superior temporal line.

The deep branches of the supratrochlear and supraorbital arteries, which supply the pericranium, and the medial branches of the supraorbital nerve, penetrate the corrugator supercilii muscle.

The scalp consists of five layers: the skin, the connective tissue, the galea (aponeurosis), the loose areolar tissue, and the pericranium. The first three layers are bound together as a single unit. This unit can move along the loose areolar tissue over the pericranium, which is adherent to the calvaria. The pericranium is the external periosteum that covers the outer surface of the skull.

The pericranial flap consists of the pericranium and loose areolar tissue. The main blood supply to the flap is from the deep branches of the supratrochlear and supraorbital vessels.

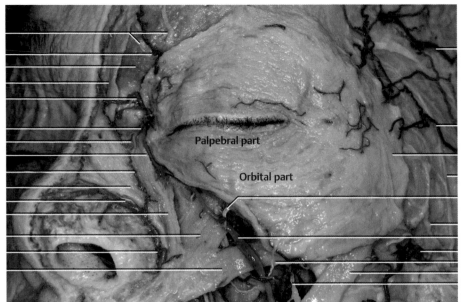

Supratrochlear n.
Supratrochlear a.
Corrugator supercilii m.
Procerus m.
Supratrochlear v.

Dorsal nasal a.
Infratrochlear n.
Angular v.
Angular a.
Nasalis m.
Nerve to nasalis m.
Levator labii superioris
alaeque nasi m.
Levator labii superioris m.
Lateral nasal a.
Zygomaticus minor m.

Palpebral part

Orbital part

Frontal br. of superficial
temporal a.

Zygomatico-orbital a.

Orbicularis oculi m.

Temporal br. of facial n.
Zygomaticobuccal br.
to orbicularis oculi m.
Upper zygomatic br.
of facial n.
Facial v.
Transverse facial a.
Inferior palpebral br.(V)
Zygomaticus major m.
Zygomaticobuccal br.
of facial n.

Fig. 5.7. The orbital region. The skin has been removed.

The temporal branch of the facial nerve does not always reach the corrugator supercilii muscle, while the zygomaticobuccal branch (see **Fig. 7.5**) usually reaches the corrugator supercilii and procerus muscles.

The lower orbicularis oculi, zygomaticus major, levator anguli oris, zygomaticus minor, risorius, levator labii superioris, levator labii superioris alaeque nasi, corrugator supercilii, procerus, nasalis, and depressor septi muscles are innervated by the zygomaticobuccal branches.

The lower orbicularis oculi muscle is generally innervated from its inferomedial side by one or two zygomaticobuccal branches.

The levator labii superioris muscle arises from the maxilla at the infraorbital rim, above the infraorbital foramen. Some of the fibers pass downward to insert into the skin overlying the upper lip. Other fibers merge with those of orbicularis oris muscle. It elevates the upper lip.

The levator labii superioris alaeque nasi muscle arises from the frontal process of the maxilla. This inserts into the skin and the greater nasal cartilage of the nose and into the skin and muscle of the upper lip. It elevates the upper lip and dilates the nostril.

The infratrochlear nerve is a branch from the nasociliary nerve. It supplies the skin over the bridge of the nose and at the medial corner of the upper eyelid. It leaves the orbit below the trochlea.

The dorsal nasal artery is one of the terminal branches of the ophthalmic artery. It accompanies the infratrochlear nerve and emerges between the trochlea of the superior oblique muscle and the medial palpebral ligament and supplies the upper part of the nose. It anastomoses with the angular artery of the facial artery.

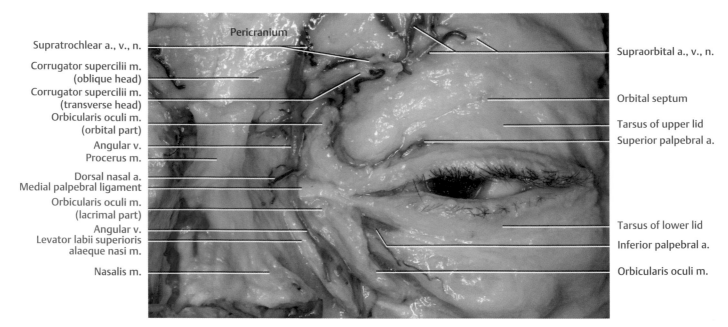

Supratrochlear a., v., n.

Corrugator supercilii m. (oblique head)

Corrugator supercilii m. (transverse head)

Orbicularis oculi m. (orbital part)

Angular v.

Procerus m.

Dorsal nasal a.

Medial palpebral ligament

Orbicularis oculi m. (lacrimal part)

Angular v.

Levator labii superioris alaeque nasi m.

Nasalis m.

Pericranium

Supraorbital a., v., n.

Orbital septum

Tarsus of upper lid

Superior palpebral a.

Tarsus of lower lid

Inferior palpebral a.

Orbicularis oculi m.

Fig. 5.8. The orbital region. The mimetic muscles have been cut and partially removed to leave their attachments.

The procerus muscle arises from the nasal bone and the upper lateral nasal cartilage and reaches into the skin between the eyebrows. It produces transverse wrinkles over the bridge of the nose.

The orbicularis oculi muscle is composed of three parts: the orbital, the palpebral, and the lacrimal. The muscle is a sphincter of the eyelids. The orbital part is the largest and arises from the nasal part of the frontal bone, the frontal process of the maxilla, and the medial palpebral ligament. The fibers pass around the orbit in concentric loops. The orbital part is involved in forced closure. The palpebral part is the central part and is confined to the eyelids. It arises from the medial palpebral ligament and runs across the eyelids to insert into the lateral palpebral ligament. The palpebral part closes the eyelids gently in involuntary or reflex blinking. The palpebral part is divided into three parts: the pretarsal, the preseptal, and the ciliary part. The lacrimal part arises from the lacrimal bone and passes behind the lacrimal sac where some fibers insert into the lacrimal fascia. The lacrimal part dilate the lacrimal sac, thereby aiding the flow of tears into the sac.

The upper orbicularis muscle is innervated by temporal branches, and the lower orbicularis muscle is innervated by the zygomatic and zygomaticobuccal branches.

The lacrimal nerve is a small branch of the ophthalmic nerve. It emerges from the upper lateral margin of the orbit to supply the lateral part of the upper eyelid.

The supraorbital, the supratrochlear, the dorsal nasal, and the superior and inferior medial palpebral arteries are the branches of the ophthalmic artery. The superior and inferior lateral palpebral arteries are the branches from the lacrimal artery. The eyelids derive their blood supply from the medial and lateral palpebral arteries. The supraorbital, supratrochlear, and angular veins form the superior ophthalmic vein in the orbit.

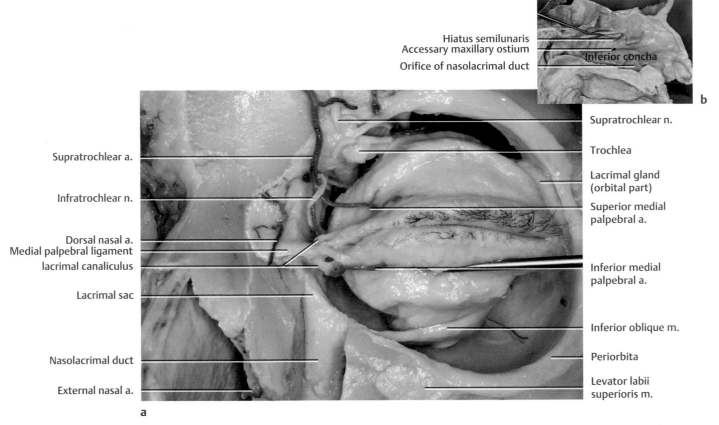

Hiatus semilunaris
Accessary maxillary ostium
Orifice of nasolacrimal duct
Inferior concha
b

Supratrochlear a.

Infratrochlear n.

Dorsal nasal a.
Medial palpebral ligament
lacrimal canaliculus

Lacrimal sac

Nasolacrimal duct

External nasal a.

Supratrochlear n.

Trochlea

Lacrimal gland
(orbital part)

Superior medial
palpebral a.

Inferior medial
palpebral a.

Inferior oblique m.

Periorbita

Levator labii
superioris m.

a

Fig. 5.9a,b. (a) The orbital region. The lacrimal apparatus has been exposed. (b) Medial view of the lateral nasal wall.

The lacrimal apparatus consists of lacrimal gland, the lacrimal canaliculi, the lacrimal sac, and the nasolacrimal duct.

The lacrimal gland is divided into two parts: orbital and palpebral. The orbital is larger and lies in a fossa in the frontal bone. The innervation of the lacrimal gland is associated with pterygopalatine ganglion. Postganglionic parasympathetic fibers pass into the maxillary nerve and run with its zygomatic branch into the orbit. They join the lacrimal nerve, derived from the ophthalmic nerve, to reach the lacrimal gland. Sensory fibers associated with the gland are derived from the lacrimal nerve.

The lacrimal sac lies adjacent to the lacrimal groove in the anterior part of the medial wall of the orbit. The sac is bounded anteriorly by the anterior lacrimal crest of the maxilla and posteriorly by the posterior lacrimal crest of the lacrimal bone.

The nasolacrimal duct passes downward from the lacrimal sac to the anterior portion of the inferior meatus on the lateral wall of the nose. The duct lies in a bony canal and produces a ridge in the medial wall of the maxillary sinus. The shape and position of the opening of the nasolacrimal duct into the inferior meatus varies (**Fig. 5.9b**).

6 Temporal Region

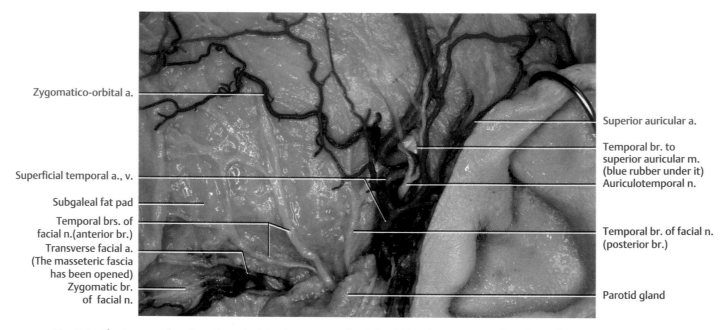

Zygomatico-orbital a.

Superficial temporal a., v.

Subgaleal fat pad

Temporal brs. of
facial n.(anterior br.)

Transverse facial a.
(The masseteric fascia
has been opened)

Zygomatic br.
of facial n.

Superior auricular a.

Temporal br. to
superior auricular m.
(blue rubber under it)
Auriculotemporal n.

Temporal br. of facial n.
(posterior br.)

Parotid gland

Fig. 6.1. The temporal region. A part of the temporoparietal fascia has been removed to show the temporal branches.

The temporal branches and communication branches are shown. The temporal branches of the facial nerve leave the parotid gland immediately inferior to the zygomatic arch. The nerve provides motor innervation to the frontalis, to the upper orbicularis oculi muscles, and occasionally, to the corrugator muscle. There are 3 to 5 temporal branches and the most auricular sided (blue rubber under it) branch innervates the superior auricular muscle. The other branches innervate the frontalis and upper orbicularis muscles.

The auriculotemporal nerve ascends on the side of the head with superficial temporal vessels. It supplies the skin of the temple and the upper part of the auricle.

The zygomatico-orbital artery is a constant branch from the superficial temporal artery to the orbicularis oculi muscle.

The superior auricular artery is a branch from the superficial temporal artery, and it runs onto the upper part of the helix.

The transverse facial artery is shown after opening the masseteric fascia. The zygomatic branches are also under this fascia and run forward with the artery.

The superficial temporal vein runs superficially on the superficial temporal artery in front of the auricle and temporal region. However, the artery runs superficially on the vein in the vertex region (see **Fig. 13.2a**).

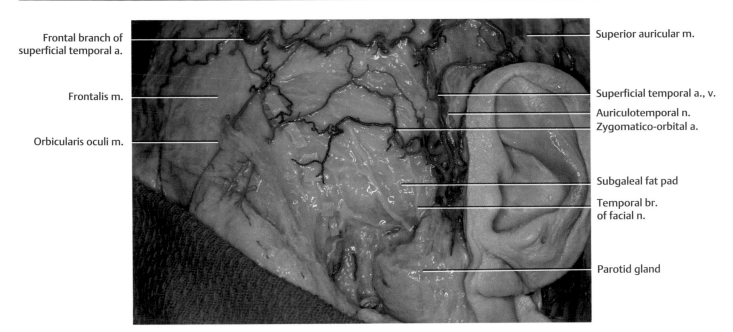

Frontal branch of
superficial temporal a.

Frontalis m.

Orbicularis oculi m.

Superior auricular m.

Superficial temporal a., v.

Auriculotemporal n.
Zygomatico-orbital a.

Subgaleal fat pad

Temporal br.
of facial n.

Parotid gland

Fig. 6.2. The temporal region. The temporal branches and their innervation to the frontalis and orbicularis oculi muscles are shown.

The temporal branches entering the frontalis muscle and the upper orbicularis oculi muscle are shown (blue rubbers under branches) after removing a part of the temporoparietal fascia. The temporal branches of the facial nerve travel in the subgaleal fat pad. The temporal branches divide into mean three rami with numerous twigs, entering deeply into the lateral end of orbicularis oculi muscle and the frontalis muscle. The temporal branches of the facial nerve generally run below the frontal branch of the superficial temporal artery.

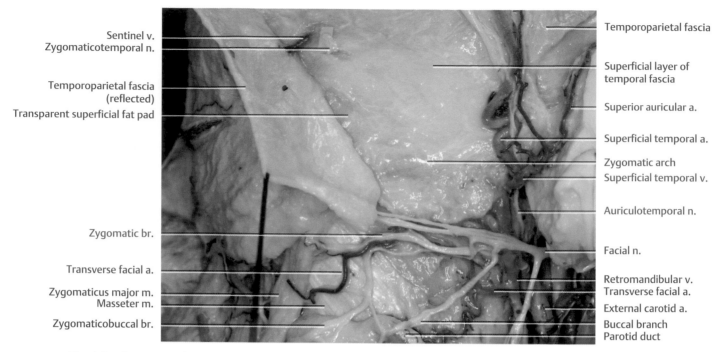

Sentinel v.
Zygomaticotemporal n.

Temporoparietal fascia
(reflected)
Transparent superficial fat pad

Zygomatic br.

Transverse facial a.

Zygomaticus major m.
Masseter m.

Zygomaticobuccal br.

Temporoparietal fascia

Superficial layer of
temporal fascia

Superior auricular a.

Superficial temporal a.

Zygomatic arch
Superficial temporal v.

Auriculotemporal n.

Facial n.

Retromandibular v.
Transverse facial a.

External carotid a.

Buccal branch
Parotid duct

Fig. 6.3. The temporal region. The temporoparietal fascia and subgaleal fat pad have been reflected anteriorly.

The "sentinel vein" is the signal for the proximity of the temporal branch of the facial nerve. The temporal branch of the facial nerve, which courses along the undersurface of the temporoparietal fascia, is generally found cephalad to the sentinel vein. This vein is located approximately 5 mm lateral to the frontozygomatic suture line and is a tributary of the internal maxillary vein draining the temporal region.

The zygomaticotemporal nerve provides sensation to the temporal skin. This nerve emerges from the orbit into the temporal fossa at approximately 14 mm inferior to the frontozygomatic suture and 10 mm lateral to the lateral margin of the orbit. This nerve is located about 1 cm lateral to the sentinel vein that passed between a perforation in the temporal fascia and the skin surface. The temporal branch of the facial nerve has a communication with the zygomaticotemporal nerve at the temporal region. The zygomaticotemporal nerve gives a branch to the lacrimal nerve in the orbit, and parasympathetic fibers that are associated with the pterygopalatine ganglion are conveyed to the lacrimal gland.

The superficial fat pad is the interfascial fat pad between the superficial and deep layer of the temporal fascia.

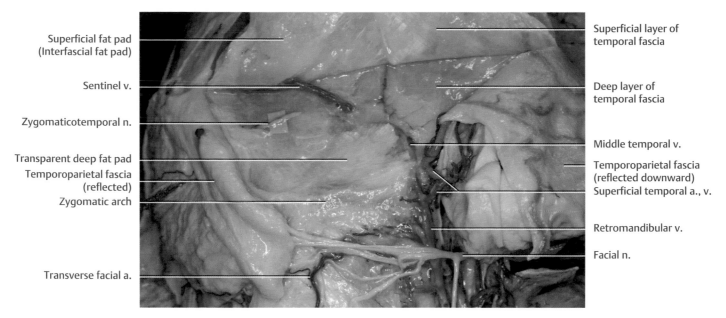

Superficial fat pad (Interfascial fat pad)

Sentinel v.

Zygomaticotemporal n.

Transparent deep fat pad
Temporoparietal fascia (reflected)
Zygomatic arch

Transverse facial a.

Superficial layer of temporal fascia

Deep layer of temporal fascia

Middle temporal v.

Temporoparietal fascia (reflected downward)
Superficial temporal a., v.

Retromandibular v.

Facial n.

Fig. 6.4. The temporal region. The superficial layer of the temporal fascia has been reflected upward.

The facial nerve branches mostly course on the lateral side of the retromandibular vein. There may be some parotid tissue between the nerve and the vein.

The sentinel vein passes backward, inferiorly and deeply, through the temporal fascia to the middle temporal vein. The middle temporal vein passes deeply on the temporalis muscle and comes up to be joined by the superficial temporal vein below the zygomatic arch to form the retromandibular vein in

the parotid gland. The retromandibular vein is joined by the maxillary vein in the parotid gland. Near the tail of the parotid gland, it usually divides into anterior and posterior branches.

The deep fat pad, which is between the temporalis muscle and the deep layer of the temporal fascia, is transparent through the deep layer of the temporal fascia. The temporal fascia splits into the superficial and the deep layer below the level of the superior orbital rim.

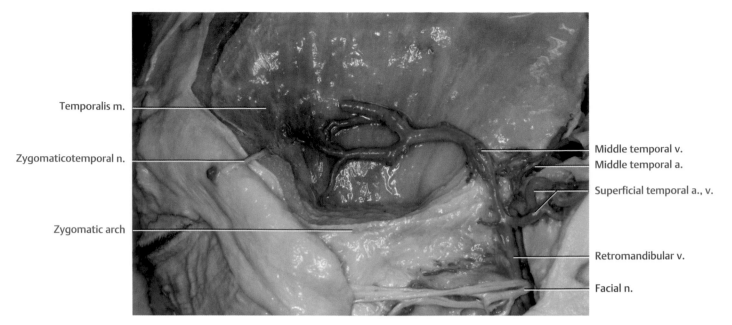

Temporalis m.

Zygomaticotemporal n.

Zygomatic arch

Middle temporal v.
Middle temporal a.

Superficial temporal a., v.

Retromandibular v.

Facial n.

Fig. 6.5. The temporal region. The deep layer of the temporal fascia and the deep fat pad have been removed.

The middle temporal artery arises from the superficial temporal artery at the level of the zygomatic arch or 1 or 2 cm below it. This artery supplies the temporal fascia and approximately 20% of the posterior and upper parts of the temporalis muscle. This artery may leave a groove on the temporal bone (see **Fig. 2.3**).

The middle temporal vein arises at approximately the same level as the middle temporal artery and accompanied it closely into the deep fascia.

The temporal fascia is attached above to the superior temporal line on the cranium. The superficial layer of the temporal fascia is attached onto the lateral border of the zygomatic arch, while the deep layer of the temporal fascia is attached onto the medial border of the arch and merges with connective tissue beneath the masseter muscle.

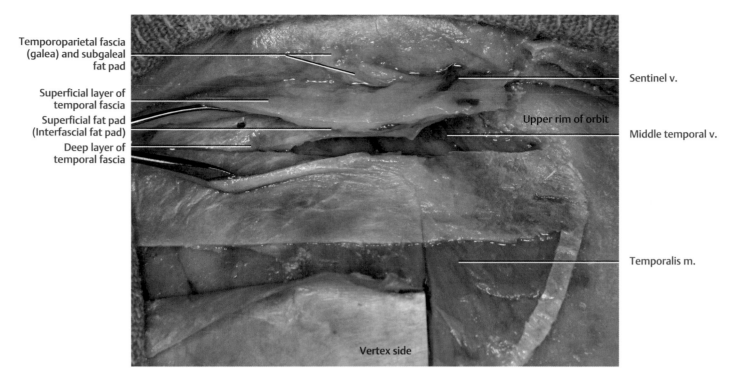

Temporoparietal fascia (galea) and subgaleal fat pad

Superficial layer of temporal fascia

Superficial fat pad (Interfascial fat pad)

Deep layer of temporal fascia

Sentinel v.

Upper rim of orbit

Middle temporal v.

Temporalis m.

Vertex side

Fig. 6.6. The temporal region. The superficial and deep layers of the temporal fascia have been separated.

The temporal branch of the facial nerve courses on the underside of the temporoparietal fascia and into the subgaleal fat pad. Several techniques in frontotemporal craniotomy preserve the temporal branch of the facial nerve. The dissection between the deep layer of the temporal fascia and the temporalis muscle is the most reliable technique for facial nerve preservation. However, postoperative temporal hollowing after the coronal approach is related to a decrease in the volume of the superficial temporal fat pad. Therefore, the better cosmetic result can be achieved by suprafascial (superficial layer of the temporal fascia) dissection.

The temporal fascia is the fascia of the temporalis muscle. The thick layer arises from the superior temporal line, where it fuses with the pericranium. The temporalis muscle arises from the deep surface of the temporal fascia and the entire temporal fossa. At the level of the upper orbital rim, the temporal fascia splits into the superficial layer and the deep layer. The former attaches to the lateral border and the latter to the medial border of the zygomatic arch. The fat pad between the superficial and deep layer of the fascia is superficial fat pad (interfascial fat pad).

There are three fat pads in the temporal region: subgaleal, superficial (interfascial), and deep.

7 Superficial Structures in the Midfacial Region

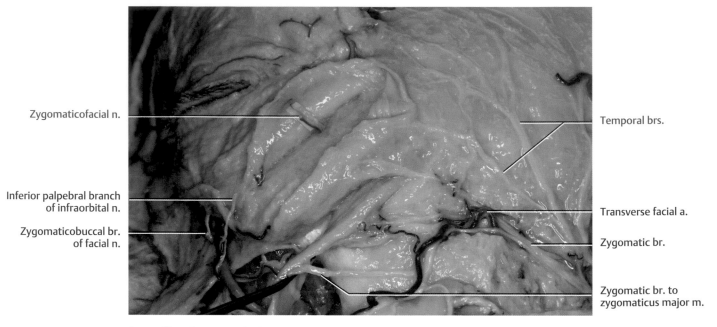

Zygomaticofacial n.

Inferior palpebral branch of infraorbital n.

Zygomaticobuccal br. of facial n.

Temporal brs.

Transverse facial a.

Zygomatic br.

Zygomatic br. to zygomaticus major m.

Fig. 7.1. The midfacial region. The lower lateral portion of the orbicularis oculi muscle has been reflected.

Innervation to the lower orbicularis oculi muscle and zygomaticus major muscle are shown. The zygomaticus major muscle is innervated by the zygomatic branches and also from the zygomaticobuccal branches (see **Fig. 7.5**) in its lower part of the muscle. The lower orbicularis muscle is innervated from its inferolateral side by one or two zygomatic branches and temporal branches.

The zygomaticofacial nerve (shown in **Fig. 7.1** with blue sheet under it) is a sensory nerve, which supplies the small region of the cheek, and it is divided from the zygomatic nerve in the orbit.

The transverse facial artery, which originates from the superficial temporal artery within the parotid gland, courses anteriorly beneath the masseteric fascia above the parotid duct.

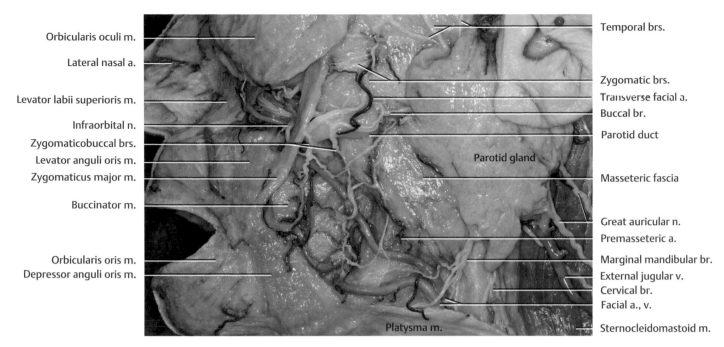

Orbicularis oculi m.

Lateral nasal a.

Levator labii superioris m.

Infraorbital n.
Zygomaticobuccal brs.
Levator anguli oris m.
Zygomaticus major m.

Buccinator m.

Orbicularis oris m.
Depressor anguli oris m.

Temporal brs.

Zygomatic brs.
Transverse facial a.
Buccal br.

Parotid duct

Parotid gland

Masseteric fascia

Great auricular n.
Premasseteric a.

Marginal mandibular br.
External jugular v.
Cervical br.
Facial a., v.

Platysma m.

Sternocleidomastoid m.

Fig. 7.2. The midfacial region.

The buccinator muscle, upper orbicularis oris muscle, and levator anguli oris muscle are innervated by the zygomaticobuccal branches (see **Fig. 7.5**). The buccinator muscle and the levator anguli oris muscle are the deep-seated muscles and they are innervated from their superficial surface.

The anterior margin of the parotid gland is a site which is suitable to identify the zygomatic and buccal branches for facial reanimation surgery. Several zygomatic and buccal branches can be exposed via the small skin incision made just below the zygomatic arch and anterior to the mandibular notch. The notch can be identified by palpation. These branches can also be exposed via preauricular skin incision. The careful selection of the donor facial nerve branches is mandatory for facial reanimation surgery because some of the buccal and zygomaticobuccal branches might not innervate the zygomaticus major muscle, which is the target muscle for smile reconstruction.

The levator anguli oris muscle arises from the canine fossa of the maxilla, immediately below the infraorbital foramen, and passes downward toward the corner of the mouth. It elevates the corner of the mouth.

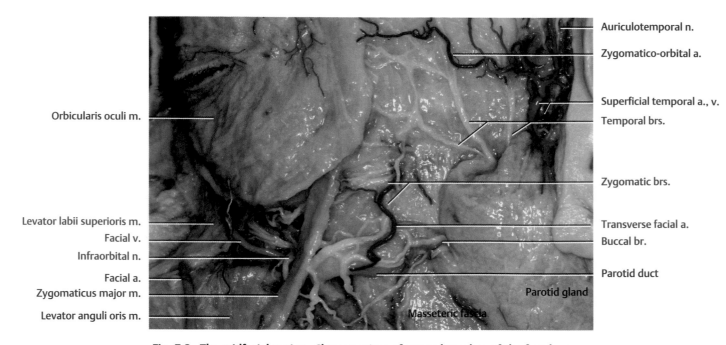

Orbicularis oculi m.

Levator labii superioris m.
Facial v.
Infraorbital n.
Facial a.
Zygomaticus major m.
Levator anguli oris m.

Auriculotemporal n.

Zygomatico-orbital a.

Superficial temporal a., v.
Temporal brs.

Zygomatic brs.

Transverse facial a.
Buccal br.

Parotid duct

Parotid gland

Masseteric fascia

Fig. 7.3. The midfacial region. Close-up view of upper branches of the facial nerve.

The facial nerve branches do not always run on the same plane. Some of the zygomatic branches run beneath the masseteric fascia anterior to the parotid gland. It is also an important surgical point that we can only divide the parotid gland just over the facial nerve branch during the dissection of the facial nerve branches in the parotid gland.

The buccal branch of the facial nerve has a close relationship with the parotid duct. The branch is most likely inferior and within 1 cm to the duct.

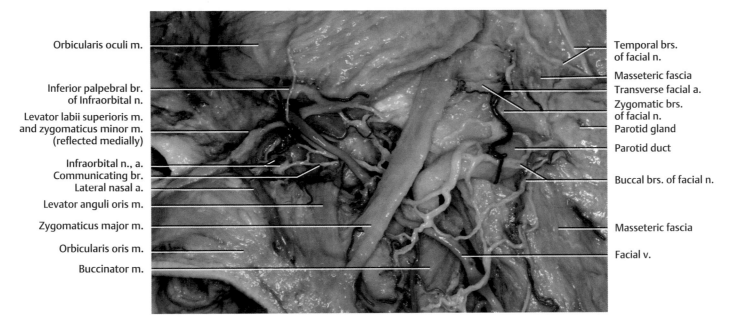

Orbicularis oculi m.

Inferior palpebral br.
of Infraorbital n.

Levator labii superioris m.
and zygomaticus minor m.
(reflected medially)

Infraorbital n., a.
Communicating br.
Lateral nasal a.

Levator anguli oris m.

Zygomaticus major m.

Orbicularis oris m.

Buccinator m.

Temporal brs.
of facial n.

Masseteric fascia

Transverse facial a.

Zygomatic brs.
of facial n.

Parotid gland

Parotid duct

Buccal brs. of facial n.

Masseteric fascia

Facial v.

Fig. 7.4. The midfacial region. Deep seated mimetic muscles and the infraorbital nerve are shown.

Some of the zygomaticobuccal branches (see **Fig. 7.5**) course downward along the parotid duct, pass under the zygomatic major muscle, then course upward to reach the lower orbicularis oculi muscle, and finally end up at the medial canthal region. The upper orbicularis oris muscle is generally innervated by the zygomaticobuccal branches. The branches reach its upper lateral side, which is medial to the zygomaticus major muscle.

The levator anguli oris and buccinator muscles are in the deepest layer of the mimetic muscles and are innervated from their superficial surface. The levator anguli oris muscle, which originated from the canine fossa, inserts into the modiolus.

The facial nerve branches have communications with the branches of the infraorbital nerve.

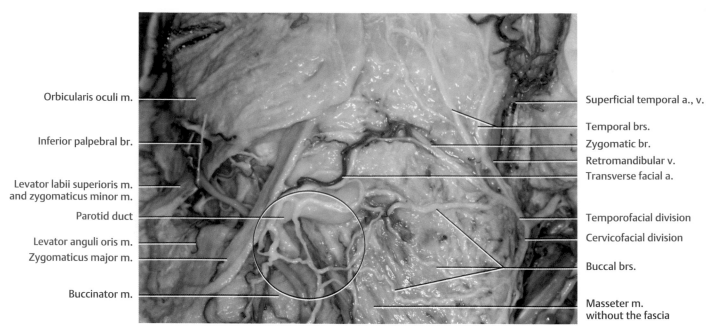

Orbicularis oculi m.

Inferior palpebral br.

Levator labii superioris m.
and zygomaticus minor m.

Parotid duct

Levator anguli oris m.

Zygomaticus major m.

Buccinator m.

Superficial temporal a., v.

Temporal brs.

Zygomatic br.

Retromandibular v.

Transverse facial a.

Temporofacial division

Cervicofacial division

Buccal brs.

Masseter m.
without the fascia

Fig. 7.5. The midfacial region. Zygomaticobuccal plexus is shown. The superficial lobe of the parotid gland has been removed.

The facial nerve divides into temporofacial (upper trunk) and cervicofacial (lower trunk) divisions just before entering the parotid gland. These divisions generally pass forward over the retromandibular vein in the parotid gland.

The facial nerve and its branches course in the parotid gland, thereby dividing the parotid gland into deep and superficial lobes. There is no anatomical plane between the lobes.

The inferior zygomatic branches usually form a zygomaticobuccal plexus (see *circled area*) with the buccal branches. The mimetic muscles (zygomaticus major, zygomaticus minor, risorius, lower orbicularis oculi, corrugator supercilii, procerus, nasalis, depressor septi, levator anguli oris, and levator labii superioris) are generally innervated by the zygomaticobuccal branches.

The zygomaticus major muscle originates from the lateral surface of the zygomatic bone, just in front of the zygomaticotemporal suture. It pulls the corner of the mouth upward and outward.

The zygomaticus minor muscle originates from the zygomatic bone just in front of the origin of zygomaticus major and runs downward and forward to insert into the upper lip. It elevates the upper lip.

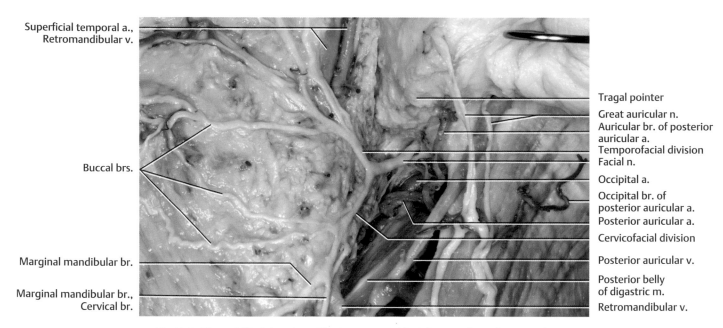

Superficial temporal a., Retromandibular v.

Buccal brs.

Marginal mandibular br.

Marginal mandibular br., Cervical br.

Tragal pointer

Great auricular n.
Auricular br. of posterior auricular a.
Temporofacial division
Facial n.

Occipital a.

Occipital br. of posterior auricular a.
Posterior auricular a.

Cervicofacial division

Posterior auricular v.

Posterior belly of digastric m.
Retromandibular v.

Fig. 7.6. The midfacial region. The intraparotid facial nerve branches are shown.

The buccal branches generally originate from both the upper and lower trunk of the facial nerve and connect with the marginal mandibular branch.

The tragal pointer or cartilage, which lies anterior to the opening of the external acoustic meatus, points directly to the facial nerve on exiting the stylomastoid foramen. The facial nerve exits about 1 cm below and medial to the tip of the tragal pointer. However, the cartilage is mobile and asymmetrical, with a blunt irregular tip, so it might be difficult to decide on the position of the tragal pointer.

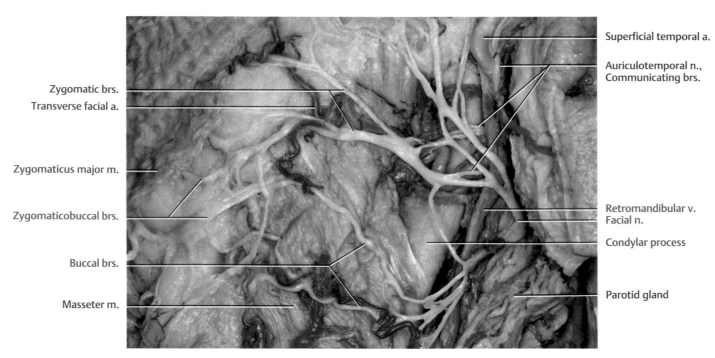

Zygomatic brs.
Transverse facial a.

Zygomaticus major m.

Zygomaticobuccal brs.

Buccal brs.

Masseter m.

Superficial temporal a.

Auriculotemporal n.,
Communicating brs.

Retromandibular v.
Facial n.

Condylar process

Parotid gland

Fig. 7.7. The midfacial region. The substance of the parotid gland has been removed.

The facial nerve communicates with the trigeminal nerve.

The auriculotemporal nerve courses from the posteromedial aspect of the neck of the mandibular condyle to an anterolateral direction to wrap around the neck of the condyle. It emerges approximately 1.5 cm below the condylar head. This nerve innervates the capsule of the temporomandibular joint. On entering the parotid gland, it turns to emerge superficially between the temporomandibular joint and external acoustic meatus. Study shows that the branches of the auriculotemporal nerve constantly communicate with the upper trunk of the facial nerve in the parotid gland. These communications might convey proprioceptive impulses from the upper facial muscles to the trigeminal nuclei of the brainstem.

The retromandibular vein in the parotid gland is a landmark for the facial nerve branches. The vein mostly courses just beneath the facial nerve.

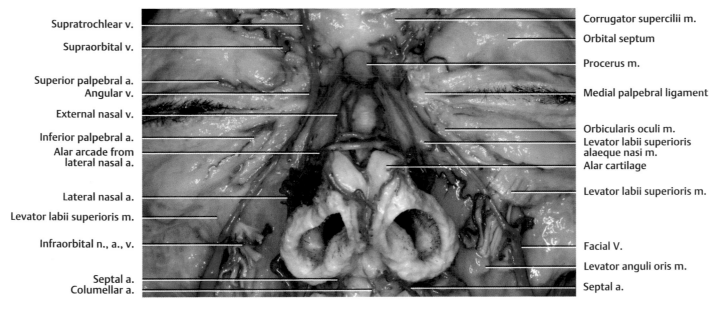

Supratrochlear v.

Supraorbital v.

Superior palpebral a.
Angular v.

External nasal v.

Inferior palpebral a.
Alar arcade from
lateral nasal a.

Lateral nasal a.

Levator labii superioris m.

Infraorbital n., a., v.

Septal a.
Columellar a.

Corrugator supercilii m.

Orbital septum

Procerus m.

Medial palpebral ligament

Orbicularis oculi m.
Levator labii superioris
alaeque nasi m.
Alar cartilage

Levator labii superioris m.

Facial V.

Levator anguli oris m.
Septal a.

Fig. 7.8. The midfacial region. The mimetic muscles have been removed to leave their attachments.

The angular vein is formed by the confluence of the supraorbital and supratrochlear veins at the medial eyelid area. The transverse supraorbital vein, which joins the supratrochlear veins on the medial side and the superficial temporal vein on the lateral side, is located in the supraorbital area (see **Fig. 5.3**). The angular vein becomes the facial vein at its junction with the superior labial vein, but the latter is not invariably present. The external nasal vein drains the external nose and empties into the angular or facial vein. The facial vein does have venous valves, particularly around the level of

the mandible. The angular vein also has valves in its tributaries. There is a communication between the facial vein and cavernous sinus via the supratrochlear and superior ophthalmic veins. The infraorbital vein links the facial vein with the pterygoid venous plexus in the infratemporal fossa (see **Fig. 10.4**).

The septal artery and columellar artery, which supplies the nasal septum and columella, generally originate from the superior labial artery. Bilateral lateral nasal arteries form the alar arcade on the dorsum of nose.

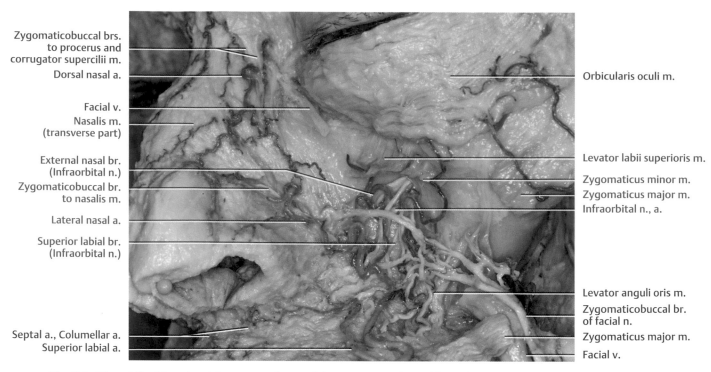

Zygomaticobuccal brs. to procerus and corrugator supercilii m.

Dorsal nasal a.

Facial v.

Nasalis m. (transverse part)

External nasal br. (Infraorbital n.)

Zygomaticobuccal br. to nasalis m.

Lateral nasal a.

Superior labial br. (Infraorbital n.)

Septal a., Columellar a.

Superior labial a.

Orbicularis oculi m.

Levator labii superioris m.

Zygomaticus minor m.

Zygomaticus major m.

Infraorbital n., a.

Levator anguli oris m.

Zygomaticobuccal br. of facial n.

Zygomaticus major m.

Facial v.

Fig. 7.9. The midfacial region. The proximal site of the zygomaticobuccal branches are cut and dislocated downward.

Innervation to the procerus, corrugator supercilii and nasalis muscles are shown. These muscles are dominantly innervated by the zygomaticobuccal branches (see **Fig. 7.5**), although the corrugator supercilii muscle might be innervated by the temporal branches of the facial nerve.

The communications between the infraorbital nerve and zygomaticobuccal branches are shown.

The facial artery bifurcates into the lateral nasal artery and superior labial artery at the angle of the mouth. After the bifurcating, the facial artery terminates as the angular artery, which communicates with the dorsal nasal artery of the ophthalmic artery.

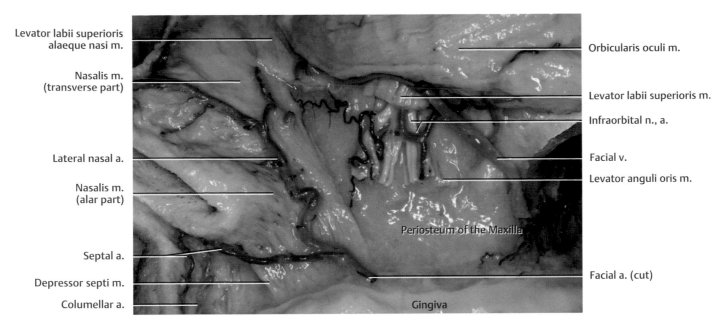

Levator labii superioris alaeque nasi m.

Nasalis m. (transverse part)

Lateral nasal a.

Nasalis m. (alar part)

Septal a.

Depressor septi m.

Columellar a.

Orbicularis oculi m.

Levator labii superioris m.

Infraorbital n., a.

Facial v.

Levator anguli oris m.

Periosteum of the Maxilla

Facial a. (cut)

Gingiva

Fig. 7.10. The midfacial region. The levator labii muscles have been removed to leave their attachments.

The nasalis muscle arises from the maxilla, overlying the root of the canine tooth (transverse part) and the lateral incisor (alar part). The transverse part of nasalis inserts into the lateral nasal cartilage and also passes over the dorsum of the nose to join the opposite side. The alar part of nasalis inserts into the greater nasal cartilage. The former compresses the nasal aperture and the latter dilate the nostril. Nasal obstruction in facial nerve paralysis is due to the nasalis muscle weakness.

The depressor septi muscle arises from the incisor region of the maxilla and passes upward from beneath the orbicularis oris muscle to insert into the nasal septum. It pulls the nasal septum downward and constricts the nostril.

The levator labii superioris muscle arises from the maxilla at the infraorbital rim, above the infraorbital foramen.

The levator anguli oris muscle arises from the canine fossa of the maxilla, immediately below the infraorbital foramen.

The infraorbital nerve emerges from the infraorbital foramen just below the origin of levator labii superioris muscle, and it divides into four branches: inferior palpebral branch, which innervates the lower eyelid skin and conjunctiva; the external nasal branch, which innervates the lateral surface of nose; the internal nasal branch, which innervates the nasal vestibule and nasal septum; and the superior labial branch, which innervates the upper lip skin and mucosa.

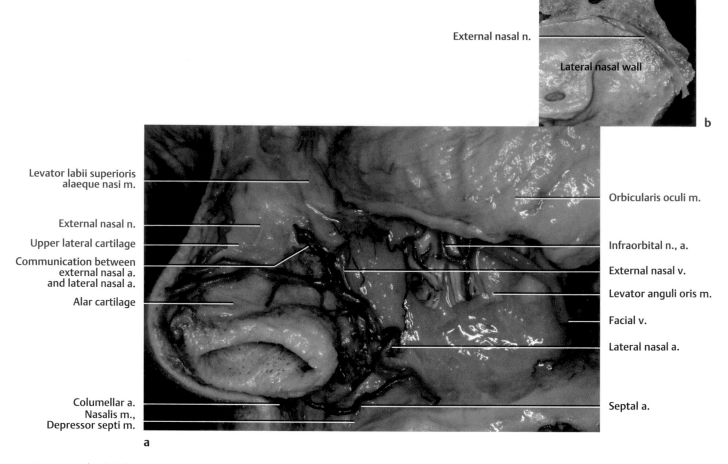

Fig. 7.11a,b. (a) The midfacial region. The nasalis and depressor septi muscles have been removed to leave their attachments, (b) Medial view of the lateral nasal wall.

The anterior ethmoidal nerve and artery enter the roof of the nasal cavity and give rise to the lateral and medial internal nasal branches. The lateral internal branches pass to the lateral wall of the nose, whereas the medial internal nasal branches run to the nasal septum. These branches supply an area in front of the nasal conchae and the anterior extremities of the middle and inferior conchae. Then, the nerve and artery run under the surface of the nasal bone (**Fig. 7.11b**) and pass between the nasal bone and the lateral nasal cartilage. When the anterior ethmoidal nerve and artery emerge at the inferior margin of the nasal bone, they become the external nasal nerve and artery. The external nasal nerve and artery supply the nasal tip, with the exception of the nasal alar region.

The lateral nasal artery or superior labial artery gives off the septal artery to the nasal septum, and the former communicates with the external nasal artery.

8 Maxillary Region

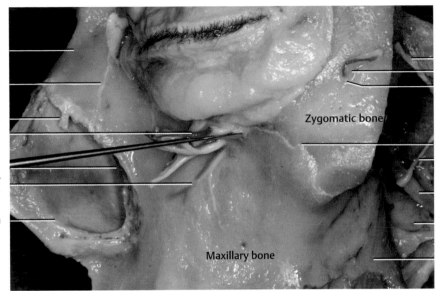

Nasal bone

Nasomaxillary suture

External nasal n.
Infraorbital n., a.

External nasal a.
Anterior superior alveolar
n., a.

Nasal septum

Deep temporal n.
Zygomaticofacial n.
Zygomaticofacial foramen

Zygomatic bone

Zygomaticomaxillary suture
Buccal n.

Maxillary a.

Lateral pterygoid plate

Maxillary bone

Maxillary tuberosity

Fig. 8.1. The maxillary region. The mimetic muscles have been removed.

The infraorbital nerve and zygomaticofacial nerve pass through each foramen respectively. The zygomaticofacial nerve supplies the skin over the prominence of the cheek.

The anterior superior alveolar nerve arises from the infraorbital nerve within the infraorbital canal and runs within the bone of the anterior maxillary wall. It supplies the anterior third of half side of teeth.

The middle superior alveolar nerve is an inconsistent branch that arises from the infraorbital nerve or maxillary nerve. It supplies the sinus mucosa, the middle third of half side of teeth when it presents. In the majority of cases, it is nonexistent, so the posterior superior alveolar nerve alone innervates the premolars and molars.

The infraorbital artery originates from the pterygopalatine segment of the maxillary artery. It enters the orbit through the inferior orbital fissure, runs on the floor of the orbit in the infraorbital groove and canal, and emerges onto the face at the infraorbital foramen.

The anterior superior alveolar artery originates from the infraorbital artery within the infraorbital canal. It supplies the anterior teeth and the anterior part of the maxillary sinus.

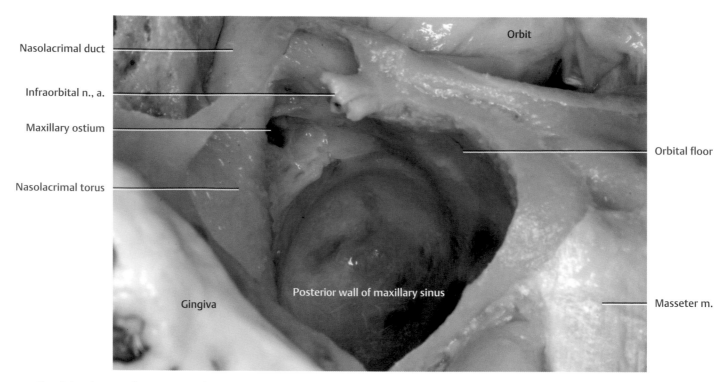

Nasolacrimal duct

Infraorbital n., a.

Maxillary ostium

Nasolacrimal torus

Orbit

Orbital floor

Posterior wall of maxillary sinus

Gingiva

Masseter m.

Fig. 8.2. The maxillary region. The anterior wall of the maxilla has been removed to expose the sinus and nasolacrimal duct.

The infraorbital nerve and vessels run on the roof of the maxillary sinus. The maxillary ostium is seen at a high position behind the nasolacrimal duct on the medial wall of the sinus. An accessory ostium is sometimes present behind the major ostium.

The innervation of the maxillary sinus is derived from the maxillary nerve via its infraorbital and anterior, middle, and posterior superior alveolar nerves.

The bony canal for the nasolacrimal duct has been partially opened to expose the nasolacrimal duct. The duct forms a bony torus on the medial wall of the maxillary sinus.

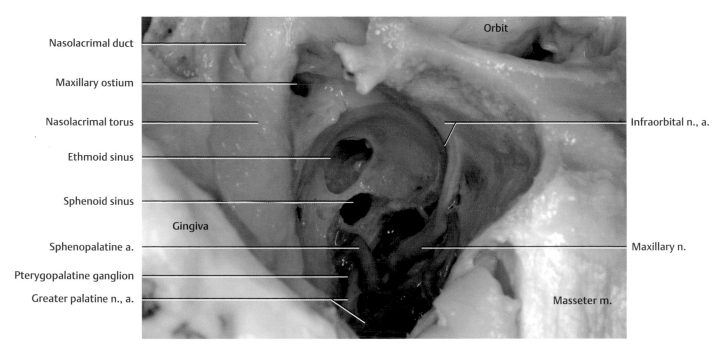

Nasolacrimal duct

Maxillary ostium

Nasolacrimal torus

Ethmoid sinus

Sphenoid sinus

Gingiva

Sphenopalatine a.

Pterygopalatine ganglion

Greater palatine n., a.

Orbit

Infraorbital n., a.

Maxillary n.

Masseter m.

Fig. 8.3. The maxillary region. The posterior and medial walls of the maxilla have been opened.

The ethmoid sinus and the sphenoid sinus have been opened through the medial maxillary wall. The infraorbital nerve and vessels are exposed by removing the bony roof of the maxillary sinus.

The sphenopalatine artery enters the lateral wall of the nose through the sphenopalatine foramen. The artery accompanies the posterior superior nasal nerve and supplies the posterior part of the lateral nasal wall before crossing the roof of the nasal cavity to accompany the nasopalatine nerve and supply the posterior-inferior part of the nasal septum.

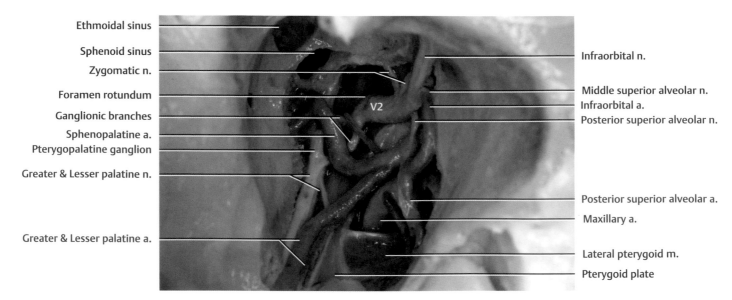

Ethmoidal sinus
Sphenoid sinus
Zygomatic n.
Foramen rotundum
Ganglionic branches
Sphenopalatine a.
Pterygopalatine ganglion
Greater & Lesser palatine n.
Greater & Lesser palatine a.

V2

Infraorbital n.
Middle superior alveolar n.
Infraorbital a.
Posterior superior alveolar n.
Posterior superior alveolar a.
Maxillary a.
Lateral pterygoid m.
Pterygoid plate

Fig. 8.4. The maxillary region. The veins have been removed.

The pterygopalatine ganglion is a parasympathetic ganglion found in the pterygopalatine fossa and largely innervated by the greater petrosal nerve. It is situated just below the maxillary nerve. The ganglionic branches, usually two in number, connect the maxillary nerve to the pterygopalatine ganglion. The pterygopalatine ganglion supplies the lacrimal gland, the paranasal sinuses, the glands of the mucosa of the nasal cavity and pharynx, the gingiva, and the mucous membrane and glands of the hard palate.

The pterygopalatine fossa contains blood vessels and nerves supplying the nose, palate, and upper jaw, including the maxillary division of the trigeminal nerve which passes through the foramen rotundum; the nerve of the pterygoid canal and accompanying vessels which pass through the pterygoid canal; the nasopalatine and posterior superior nasal nerves and the sphenopalatine vessels which pass through the sphenopalatine foramen; the greater and lesser palatine nerves, which together with accompanying vessels pass through the greater and lesser palatine foramina. The pharyngeal branch of the pterygopalatine ganglion runs through the palatovaginal canal to supply the nasopharyngeal mucosa.

The nasopalatine nerve and sphenopalatine vessels run into the nasal cavity through the sphenopalatine foramen, and they pass across the roof of the nasal cavity to reach the nasal septum and supply the posteroinferior part of the nasal septum.

The zygomatic nerve arises in the pterygopalatine fossa from the maxillary nerve. It enters the orbit by the inferior orbital fissure and divides at the back of that cavity into two branches, the zygomaticotemporal nerve and the zygomaticofacial nerve. The zygomatic nerve carries sensory fibers from the skin. It also carries postsynaptic parasympathetic fibers (originating in the pterygopalatine ganglion) to the lacrimal nerve via a communication. These fibers will eventually provide innervation to the lacrimal gland. These parasympathetic postganglionic fibers come from the facial nerve.

The third segment of the maxillary artery is the pterygopalatine segment. It has five branches: the posterior superior alveolar artery, the infraorbital artery, the artery of the pterygoid canal, the descending palatine artery, and the sphenopalatine artery.

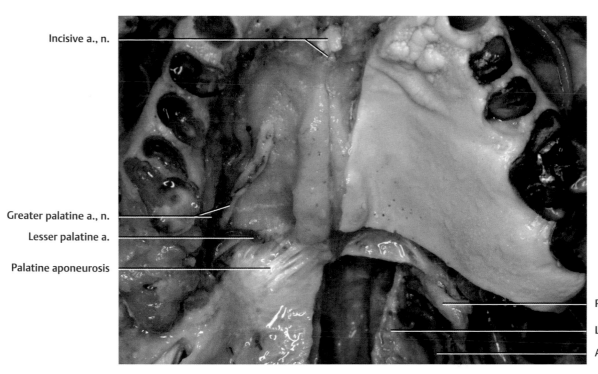

Incisive a., n.

Greater palatine a., n.

Lesser palatine a.

Palatine aponeurosis

Pterygoid hamulus

Levator veli palatini m.

Ascending palatine a.

Fig. 8.5. The palatal region. The palatal mucosa has been removed on the right side and the soft palate has been removed on the left side.

The greater and lesser palatine nerves and arteries pass from the pterygopalatine fossa down the greater palatine canal at the back of the lateral wall of the nose. The greater palatine nerve and artery run through the greater palatine foramen and onto the back of the hard palate. They pass toward the front of the hard palate. They supply the palatal mucosa and palatal gingiva. Within the greater palatine canal, the nerve and artery give off nasal branches that innervate the posteroinferior part of the lateral wall of the nasal cavity.

The lesser palatine nerve and artery emerge onto the palate at the lesser palatine foramen. They run backward into the soft palate.

The nasopalatine nerve terminates as the incisive nerve which passes through the incisive canal with an accompany artery onto the hard palate to supply oral mucosa around the incisive papilla. It communicates with the corresponding nerve of the opposite side and with the greater palatine nerve.

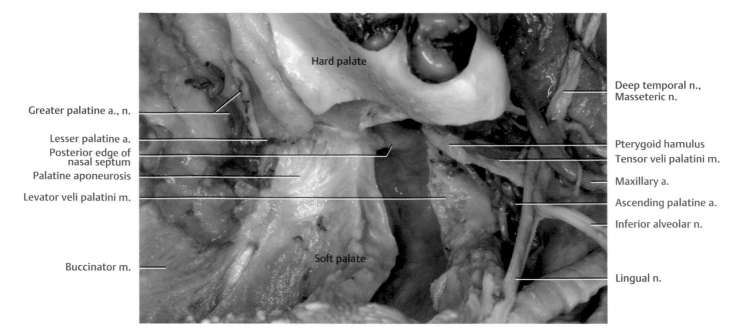

Greater palatine a., n.

Lesser palatine a.
Posterior edge of nasal septum
Palatine aponeurosis

Levator veli palatini m.

Buccinator m.

Hard palate

Soft palate

Deep temporal n., Masseteric n.

Pterygoid hamulus
Tensor veli palatini m.

Maxillary a.

Ascending palatine a.

Inferior alveolar n.

Lingual n.

Fig. 8.6. The palatal region. The levator and tensor veli palatini muscles are shown on the left side.

The tensor veli palatini muscle arises from the scaphoid fossa of the sphenoid bone (at the root of the pterygoid plate) and from the lateral side of the cartilaginous part of the Eustachian tube. The fibers converge toward the pterygoid hamulus, where the muscle becomes tendinous. The tendon bends at right angles around the hamulus to become the palatine aponeurosis. The aponeurosis is attached to the posterior border of the hard palate. This muscle pulls the soft palate laterally. This muscle is innervated by the branch of the mandibular nerve via the nerve to the medial pterygoid muscle.

The levator veli palatini muscle originates from the base of the skull at the apex of the petrous part of the temporal bone and from the medial side of the cartilaginous part of the Eustachian tube. The muscle curves downward, medially, and forward to enter the palate immediately below the opening of the Eustachian tube. This muscle produces upward and backward movement of the soft palate. This muscle is innervated by the accessory nerve via the pharyngeal plexus.

The ascending palatine artery originates from the facial artery in the neck. It divides near the levator veli palatini muscle into two branches. One supplies and follows the course of this muscle and, winding over the upper border of the superior pharyngeal constrictor, supplies the soft palate and the palatine glands. The other pierces the superior pharyngeal constrictor and supplies the palatine tonsil and auditory tube, anastomosing with the tonsillar branch of the facial artery and the ascending pharyngeal artery.

9 Masseteric Region

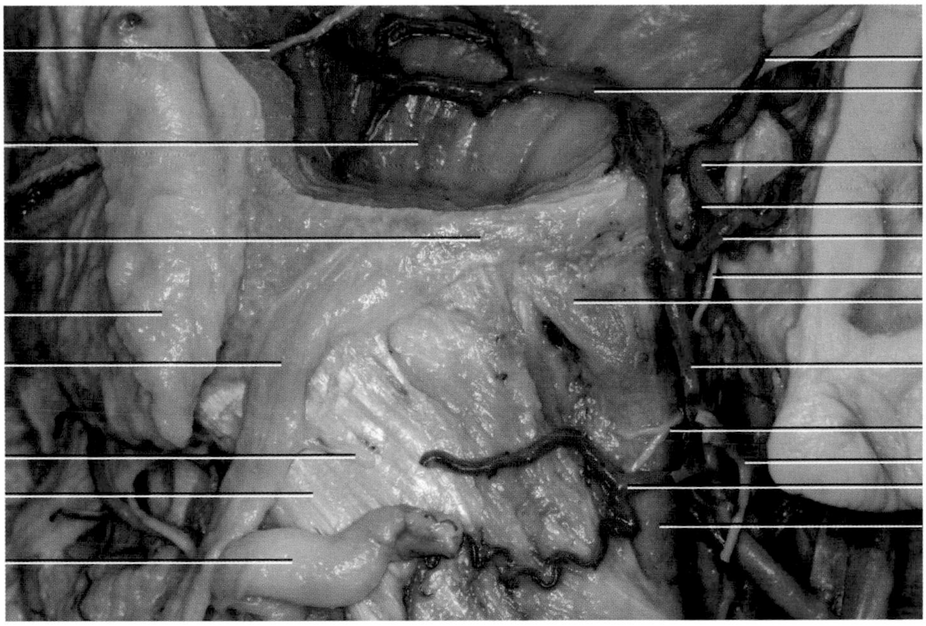

Zygomaticotemporal n.

Temporalis m.

Zygomatic arch

Orbicularis oculi m. (reflected)

Zygomaticus major m.

Muscle br.

Masseter m.

Parotid duct

Middle temporal a.
Middle temporal v.

Superficial temporal a.

Middle temporal a.
Superficial temporal v.

Auriculotemporal n.
Lateral ligament

Retromandibular v.

Auriculotemporal n.
Facial n.
Transverse facial a.

Mandibular condyle

Fig. 9.1. The masseteric region. The parotid gland and the facial nerve branches have been removed.

The zygomaticus major muscle, the masseter muscle, and the temporal fascia and lateral ligament are the structures which are attached to the zygomatic arch.

The origin of the zygomaticus major muscle is the subzygomatic fossa, which is located posterior and inferior to the malar eminence and anterior to the zygomaticotemporal suture. The subzygomatic fossa is usually an easily palpable landmark.

The retromandibular vein usually divides into anterior and posterior branches near the tail of the parotid gland. Outside the gland, anterior branch joins the facial vein to form the common facial vein, while the posterior branch unites with the posterior auricular vein to form the external jugular vein. The common facial vein drains into the internal jugular vein (see **Fig. 11.2** and **Fig. 12.3**).

The temporomandibular joint has one major ligament, the temporomandibular ligament, also termed the lateral ligament, which is actually the thickened lateral portion of the capsule. It has two parts: an outer oblique portion and an inner horizontal portion. The base of this triangular ligament is attached to the zygomatic process of the temporal bone and the articular tubercle. Its apex is fixed to the lateral side of the neck of the mandible.

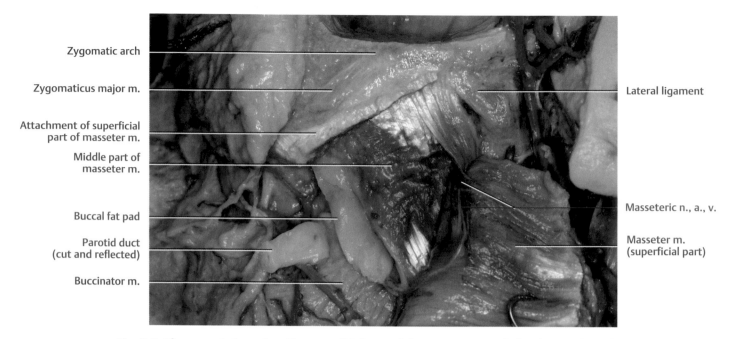

Zygomatic arch

Zygomaticus major m.

Attachment of superficial part of masseter m.

Middle part of masseter m.

Buccal fat pad

Parotid duct (cut and reflected)

Buccinator m.

Lateral ligament

Masseteric n., a., v.

Masseter m. (superficial part)

Fig. 9.2. The masseteric region. The superficial part of the masseter muscle has been reflected.

The masseter muscle is one of the muscles of mastication. It is quadrilateral in shape and consists of three layers. The layers are fused anteriorly, but diverge posteriorly. The most pronounced layer is superficial. It originates from the anterior two-thirds of the inferior border of the zygomatic arch up to the zygomatic process of the maxilla. Initially, it is aponeurotic and passes obliquely in an inferomedial direction. It inserts into the inferior border of the external surface of the angle of the mandible. Its insertion extends anteriorly to the junction of the ramus with the body of the mandible.

The chief muscles of mastication are the temporalis, masseter, medial pterygoid, and lateral pterygoid. The first three muscles raise the mandible against the maxilla with great force. The lateral pterygoid muscle assists in opening the mouth, but its main action is to draw forward the condyle and articular disk so that the mandible is protruded and the inferior incisors projected in front of the upper. In this action, it is assisted by the medial pterygoid muscle. The mandible is retracted by the posterior fibers of the temporalis muscle. The medial and lateral pterygoid muscle of two sides contract alternately to produce side-to-side movement of the mandible.

The transfer of functional innervated musculature into the face offers the possibility of meaningful facial movement. And the temporalis, masseter, and digastric muscles can be used for facial reanimation.

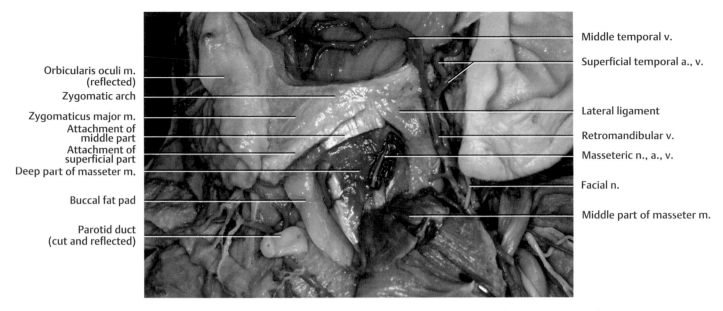

Fig. 9.3. The masseteric region. The middle part of the masseter muscle has been reflected.

The masseteric nerve and vessels course anteroinferiorly on the deep part of the masseter muscle after passing the mandibular notch.

The middle part of masseter muscle originates from the middle third of the zygomatic arch. It blends with the superficial part at the mandibular insertion and anteriorly. The posterior divergence of fibers between the superficial and deep parts of masseter muscle permits the entry of its blood supply—the masseteric artery—which is a branch of the maxillary artery. The deep part of masseter muscle has a similar course to the middle part but is separated from it by the masseteric nerve. Similar to the artery, the nerve enters posteriorly where the layers diverge.

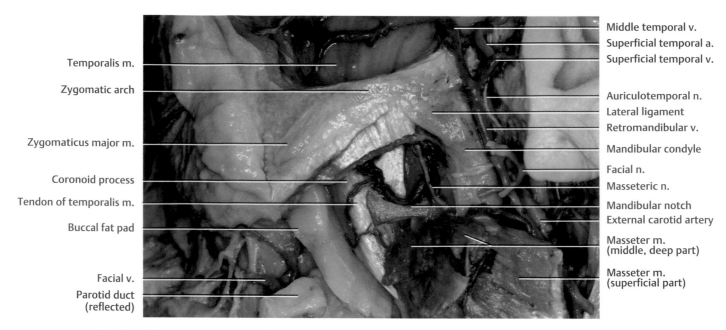

Temporalis m.

Zygomatic arch

Zygomaticus major m.

Coronoid process

Tendon of temporalis m.

Buccal fat pad

Facial v.

Parotid duct
(reflected)

Middle temporal v.

Superficial temporal a.

Superficial temporal v.

Auriculotemporal n.

Lateral ligament

Retromandibular v.

Mandibular condyle

Facial n.

Masseteric n.

Mandibular notch

External carotid artery

Masseter m.
(middle, deep part)

Masseter m.
(superficial part)

Fig. 9.4. The masseteric region. The every part of the masseter muscle has been reflected downward.

The upper border of the ramus of mandible is thin and is surmounted by two processes, the coronoid process anteriorly and the condylar process posteriorly. These are separated by a deep concavity, the mandibular notch, or sigmoid notch. It allows the passage of the masseteric nerve, the masseteric artery, and the masseteric vein.

The masseteric nerve leaves the infratemporal fossa through the mandibular notch. At this level, the nerve usually consists of one or more branches. Several intraoperative landmarks can be used to identify the masseteric nerve. The mandibular notch is a palpable and reliable bony landmark for identifying the masseteric nerve, which is located just above the notch on the deep part of the masseter muscle. The masseteric nerve is a potential source of axons for facial reinnervation when the proximal facial nerve stump is not available but the distal facial nerve and facial musculature are present and functional.

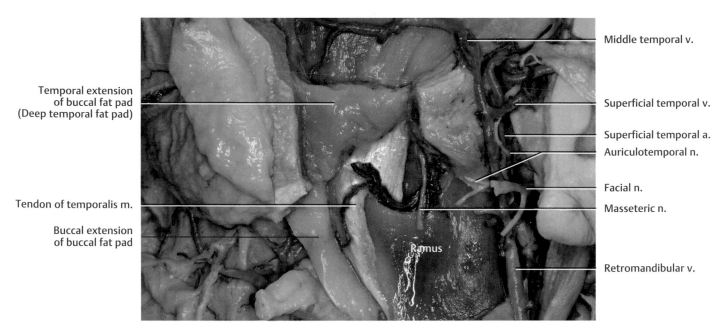

Fig. 9.5. The masseteric region. The zygomatic arch has been removed and the deep temporal fat pad preserved.

The buccal fat pad is located superficial to the buccinator muscle at the anterior edge of the masseter muscle and provides fullness to the cheek inferior to the malar prominence. It has three main extensions: buccal, pterygoid, and temporal. These extensions are each contained within a separate capsule. The proposed function is to provide a surface for the gliding motion of the muscles of mastication. The temporal extension of the buccal fat pad is identical to the deep temporal fat pad, which is situated between the temporalis muscle and the deep layer of the temporal fascia.

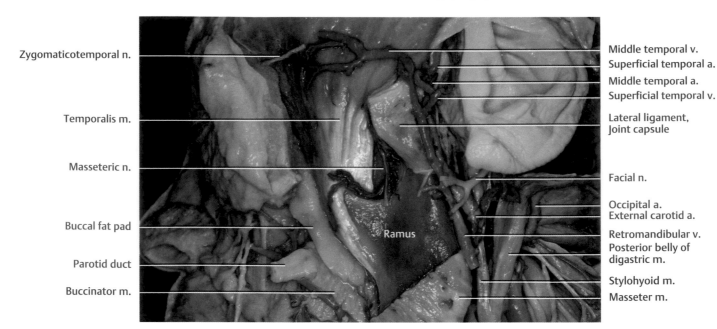

Zygomaticotemporal n.

Temporalis m.

Masseteric n.

Buccal fat pad

Parotid duct

Buccinator m.

Middle temporal v.
Superficial temporal a.

Middle temporal a.
Superficial temporal v.

Lateral ligament,
Joint capsule

Facial n.

Occipital a.
External carotid a.

Retromandibular v.
Posterior belly of
digastric m.

Stylohyoid m.
Masseter m.

Ramus

Fig. 9.6. The masseteric region. The deep temporal fat pad has been removed.

The temporalis muscle arises from the floor of the temporal fossa and from the overlying temporal fascia. The fibers converge toward their insertion onto the apex, the anterior and posterior borders, and the medial surface of the coronoid process, and the anterior border of the ramus almost as far as the third molar tooth. Many of the fibers have a tendinous insertion. The anterior (vertical) fibers of the temporalis muscle elevate the mandible; the posterior (horizontal) fibers retract it.

The temporalis muscle is an alternative muscle for reanimation of the smile. It serves as a static support to the oral commissure and provides trigeminally controlled dynamic movement.

The middle temporal artery, which is a branch of the superficial temporal artery, arises immediately above the zygomatic arch, and, perforating the temporal fascia, gives branches to the temporalis muscle, anastomosing with the deep temporal artery. It supplies the posterior part and the upper part of the temporalis muscle.

10 Deep Structures in the Midfacial Region

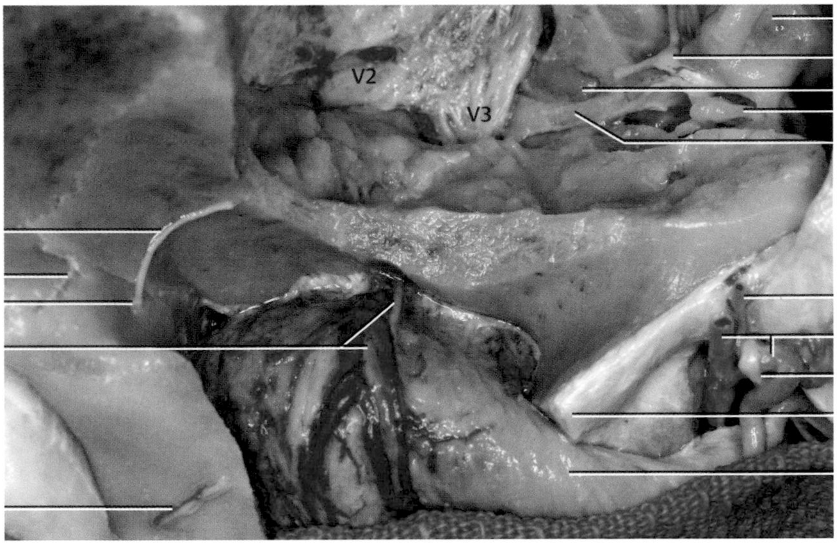

Semicircular canal
Geniculate ganglion (GSPN cut)
Internal carotid a.
Incus
Tensor tympani m.

Zygomaticotemporal n.

Frontozygomatic suture
Zygomaticotemporal foramen

Deep temporal n., a., v.

Middle temporal a.
Superficial temporal a., v.
Auriculotemporal n.
Root of zygomatic arch

Temporalis m. (reflected)

Zygomaticofacial n.

V2

V3

Fig. 10.1. Superior view of the middle fossa and temporal fossa.

The neurovascular bundle is shown on the deep surface of the temporalis muscle. The dissection of the muscle from the temporal bone might cause the muscle to atrophy because of damage to its motor nerves.

The zygomaticotemporal nerve is a terminal branch of the maxillary division of the trigeminal nerve. The zygomatic nerve enters the orbit through the inferior orbital fissure, and it divides into the zygomaticotemporal and zygomaticofacial nerves along the lateral wall of the orbit. The zygomaticotemporal nerve emerges from the orbit into the temporal fossa at approximately 14 mm inferior to the frontozygomatic suture and 10 mm lateral to the lateral margin of the orbit through the zygomaticotemporal foramen. Then, it passes through the temporalis muscle and pierces the temporal fascia about 2 cm above the zygomatic arch. The foramen is always found posterolateral to the edge of the lateral orbital rim. It is a sensory nerve that provides sensation to the skin of the temporal region.

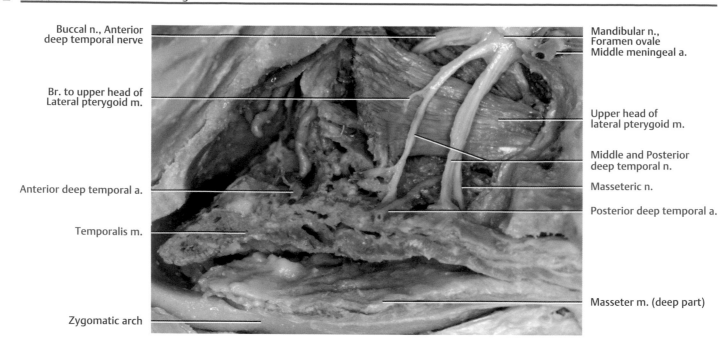

Buccal n., Anterior
deep temporal nerve

Br. to upper head of
Lateral pterygoid m.

Anterior deep temporal a.

Temporalis m.

Zygomatic arch

Mandibular n.,
Foramen ovale
Middle meningeal a.

Upper head of
lateral pterygoid m.

Middle and Posterior
deep temporal n.

Masseteric n.

Posterior deep temporal a.

Masseter m. (deep part)

Fig. 10.2. Superior view of the middle fossa without bone.

The buccal nerve and the anterior deep temporal nerve generally pass between the upper and lower heads of the lateral pterygoid muscle. The middle and posterior deep temporal nerve and masseteric nerve run on the superior surface of the upper head.

The temporalis muscle is innervated predominantly by the deep temporal nerves, which are branches of the anterior trunk of the mandibular nerve. The number of the deep temporal nerves generally vary from one to five. The temporal branches, which innervate the temporalis muscle, also arise from the buccal nerve and the masseteric nerve. They innervate the anterior and posterior part of the temporalis muscle respectively.

Three main arteries supply the temporalis muscle: the anterior deep temporal, the posterior deep temporal, and the middle temporal. The anterior deep temporal artery, which arises from the pterygoid segment of the internal maxillary artery, enters the anterior portion of the muscle and supplies about 30% of the muscle. The posterior deep temporal artery, which arises from the same segment of the maxillary artery, enters the central part of the muscle and supplies about 50% of the muscle. The middle temporal artery. which arises from the superficial temporal artery, supplies the temporal fascia and approximately 20% of the posterior and upper parts of the temporalis muscle.

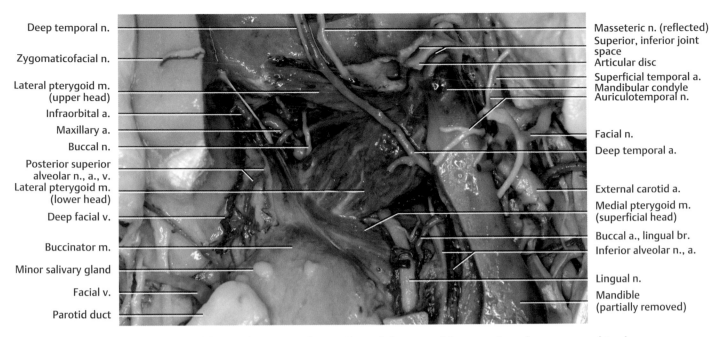

Deep temporal n.
Zygomaticofacial n.
Lateral pterygoid m. (upper head)
Infraorbital a.
Maxillary a.
Buccal n.
Posterior superior alveolar n., a., v.
Lateral pterygoid m. (lower head)
Deep facial v.
Buccinator m.
Minor salivary gland
Facial v.
Parotid duct

Masseteric n. (reflected)
Superior, inferior joint space
Articular disc
Superficial temporal a.
Mandibular condyle
Auriculotemporal n.
Facial n.
Deep temporal a.
External carotid a.
Medial pterygoid m. (superficial head)
Buccal a., lingual br.
Inferior alveolar n., a.
Lingual n.
Mandible (partially removed)

Fig. 10.3. Infratemporal fossa. The temporalis muscle and the coronoid process have been removed to show the infratemporal fossa.

The lingual nerve is a branch of the posterior trunk of the mandibular nerve. It is essentially a sensory nerve. It emerges from the inferior border of the lateral pterygoid muscle and curves downward and forward in the space between the ramus of the mandible and the medial pterygoid muscle.

The maxillary artery is a terminal branch of the external carotid artery. It arises at the posterior border of the mandibular neck. It is divided into three segments. The first is the mandibular segment, which lies behind the mandible and courses horizontally between the neck of the mandible and lateral to the sphenomandibular ligament. This segment has five branches and all enter bone, where the segment lies parallel to and a little below the auriculotemporal nerve. It crosses the inferior alveolar nerve and runs along the lower border of the lateral pterygoid muscle. These branches include the deep auricular artery, the anterior tympanic artery, the

middle meningeal artery, an accessory meningeal artery, and the inferior alveolar artery.

The inferior alveolar artery and vein descend downward and forward to join the inferior alveolar nerve. They descend to the mandibular foramen on the medial surface of the ramus of the mandible and run along the mandibular canal in the substance of the bone. Opposite the first premolar tooth, they divide into two branches: incisor and mental.

The temporomandibular joint (TMJ) is formed by the condyle of the mandible articulating in the mandibular fossa (glenoid fossa) of the temporal bone. The joint cavity is divided into two by an intra-articular disc. Its margins merge with the joint capsule. The TMJ is basically a hinge joint, but it also allows for some gliding movements. Sensory innervation of the temporomandibular joint is derived from the auriculotemporal nerve and the articular branch from the masseteric nerve.

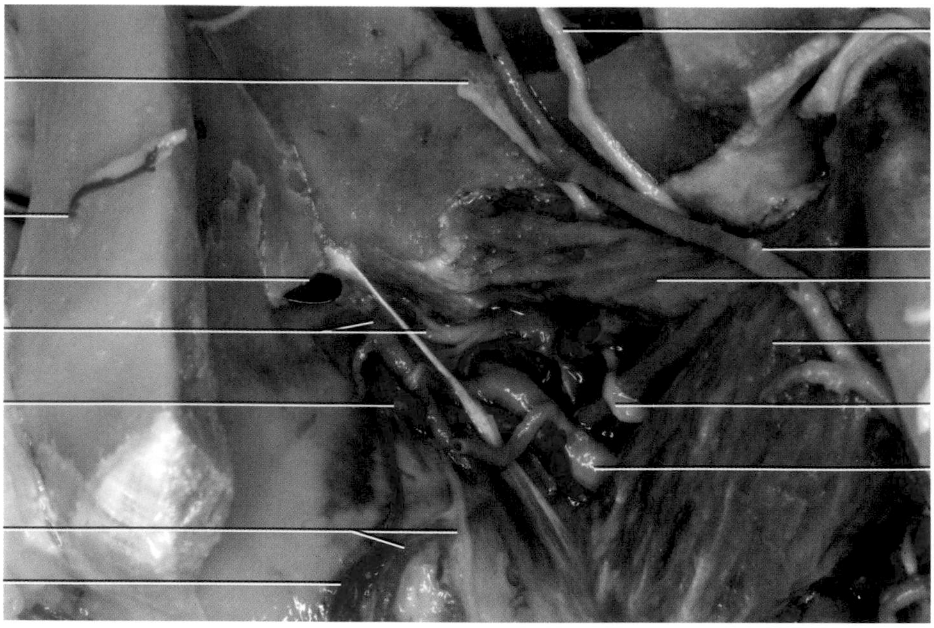

Deep temporal n.

Zygomaticofacial n.

Inferior orbital fissure

Infraorbital a., n.

Maxillary v.

Posterior superior
alveolar n., a., v.

Deep facial v.

Masseteric n. (reflected)

Deep temporal a.

Lateral pterygoid m.
(upper head)

Lateral pterygoid m.
(lower head)

Buccal n.

Maxillary a.

Fig. 10.4. Infratemporal fossa. The probe is passing through the inferior orbital fissure.

The lateral pterygoid muscle runs in the horizontal plane and occupies most of the infratemporal fossa. It has two distinct heads: a smaller upper infratemporal head and a lower pterygoid one. The infratemporal head originates at the lateral surface of the greater sphenoid wing and the infratemporal crest of the sphenoid bone. It runs parallel to the floor of the middle cranial fossa and merges posteriorly with the pterygoid head. The pterygoid head originates from the lateral surface of the lateral pterygoid plate and runs laterally and superiorly. Both heads were inserted in a depression at the anterior aspect of the neck of the mandible. The muscle assists in opening the jaws by pulling forward the mandibular condyle and the articular disc of the temporomandibular joint. The muscle is innervated by the mandibular nerve.

The posterior superior alveolar artery arises from the maxillary artery (pterygopalatine segment), frequently in conjunction with the infraorbital artery just as the maxillary artery is passing into the pterygopalatine fossa. It runs onto the maxillary tuberosity and supplies the maxillary molar and premolar teeth through the alveolar canal (see **Fig. 10.13b**), the buccal gingiva, and the maxillary air sinus. The posterior superior alveolar vein drains into the pterygoid venous plexus or the maxillary vein.

The inferior orbital fissure transmits the maxillary nerve and its zygomatic branch, the infraorbital vessels, the ascending branches from the pterygopalatine ganglion, and a vein that connects the inferior ophthalmic vein with the pterygoid venous plexus. The orbitalis muscle (Müller's muscle) occupies the lateral part of the inferior orbital fissure and forms a lamina of smooth muscle fibers that cover the inferior orbital fissure. The orbitalis muscle is a rudimentary smooth muscle that crosses from the infraorbital groove and sphenomaxillary fissure and is intimately united with the periosteum of the orbit. It lies at the back of the orbit and spans the infraorbital fissure.

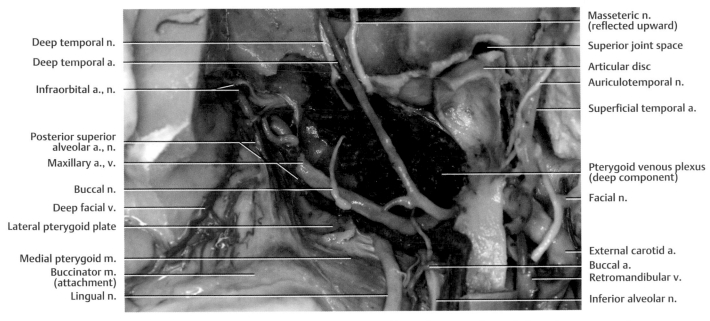

Deep temporal n.

Deep temporal a.

Infraorbital a., n.

Posterior superior alveolar a., n.

Maxillary a., v.

Buccal n.

Deep facial v.

Lateral pterygoid plate

Medial pterygoid m.

Buccinator m. (attachment)

Lingual n.

Masseteric n. (reflected upward)

Superior joint space

Articular disc

Auriculotemporal n.

Superficial temporal a.

Pterygoid venous plexus (deep component)

Facial n.

External carotid a.

Buccal a.

Retromandibular v.

Inferior alveolar n.

Fig. 10.5. Infratemporal fossa. The mandibular condyle and lateral pterygoid muscle have been removed.

The medial pterygoid muscle originates in the pterygoid fossa from the medial surface of the lateral pterygoid plate. Its fibers pass inferiorly to attach to the medial surface of the ramus and angle of the mandible. It elevates the mandible.

The pterygoid segment, which is the second segment of the maxillary artery, is related to the pterygoid head of the lateral pterygoid muscle. It runs between the infratemporal and pterygoid heads of the lateral pterygoid muscle or laterally to the pterygoid head of the lateral pterygoid muscle. It has five branches: the deep temporal arteries (anterior and posterior), the pterygoid artery, the masseteric artery, the buccal artery, and a small lingual branch.

The pterygoid venous plexus has superficial and deep components. The latter is more prominent and is located between the lateral and medial pterygoid muscles, posterior to the lateral pterygoid plate, around the lingual and inferior alveolar nerves. It communicates with the cavernous sinus, the facial vein, the retromandibular vein, the inferior ophthalmic vein, and the pharyngeal plexus. The primary drainage of the pterygoid venous plexus is posteriorly through the retromandibular vein via the maxillary vein. The deep facial vein connects the facial vein with the pterygoid venous plexus in the infratemporal fossa.

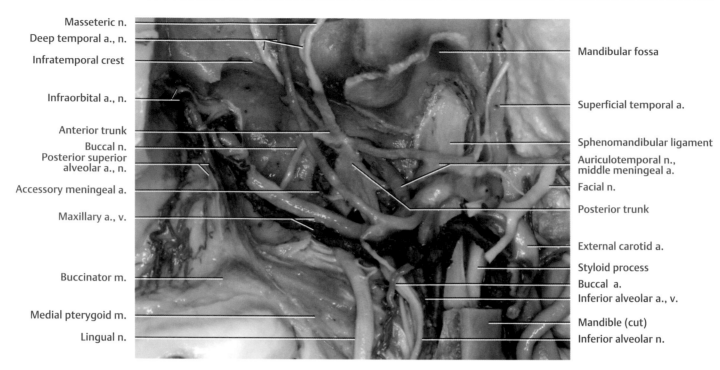

Masseteric n.
Deep temporal a., n.
Infratemporal crest

Infraorbital a., n.

Anterior trunk
Buccal n.
Posterior superior
alveolar a., n.
Accessory meningeal a.

Maxillary a., v.

Buccinator m.

Medial pterygoid m.
Lingual n.

Mandibular fossa

Superficial temporal a.

Sphenomandibular ligament
Auriculotemporal n.,
middle meningeal a.
Facial n.

Posterior trunk

External carotid a.

Styloid process
Buccal a.
Inferior alveolar a., v.

Mandible (cut)
Inferior alveolar n.

Fig. 10.6. Infratemporal fossa. The pterygoid venous plexus has been removed.

The auriculotemporal nerve originates from the posterior trunk of the mandibular nerve primarily in one or two branches. The middle meningeal artery is encircled by them in the latter. The two branches then converge to form a single nerve. This nerve is essentially sensory but it also distributes autonomic fibers to the parotid gland. The auriculotemporal nerve crosses medially to the neck of the mandible and changes its direction upward in the parotid gland between the temporomandibular joint and the external acoustic meatus.

The infratemporal fossa is the anatomic space under the floor of the middle cranial fossa and posterior to the maxilla.

The roof is the infratemporal surface of the greater sphenoid wing. The medial wall is the lateral pterygoid plate anteriorly and the tensor veli palatine and medial pterygoid muscles posteriorly. The anterior wall is the posterior surface of the maxilla. The fossa extends posteriorly to the glenoid fossa and the temporomandibular joint. Superiorly and laterally, the fossa blends into the temporal fossa and the belly of the temporalis muscle. The infratemporal crest is a transverse ridge of the greater sphenoid wing that separates the temporal fossa from the infratemporal fossa. The inferior boundary of the fossa is open.

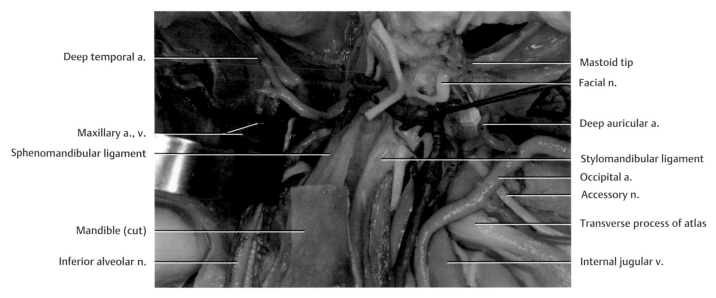

Deep temporal a.

Maxillary a., v.

Sphenomandibular ligament

Mandible (cut)

Inferior alveolar n.

Mastoid tip

Facial n.

Deep auricular a.

Stylomandibular ligament

Occipital a.

Accessory n.

Transverse process of atlas

Internal jugular v.

Fig. 10.7. Infratemporal fossa. The accessory ligaments of the temporomandibular ligament.

The accessory ligaments of the temporomandibular ligament are the stylomandibular ligament, the sphenomandibular ligament, and the pterygomandibular raphe (ligament). The stylomandibular ligament extends from the tip of the styloid process and from the styloid ligament to the angle of the mandible. The sphenomandibular ligament attaches to the spine of the sphenoid bone and descends to the lingula near the mandibular foramen in the medial surface of the ramus of the mandible. The deep auricular artery is the first branch from the mandibular segment of the maxillary artery. It supply the skin of the external acoustic meatus and part of the tympanic membrane.

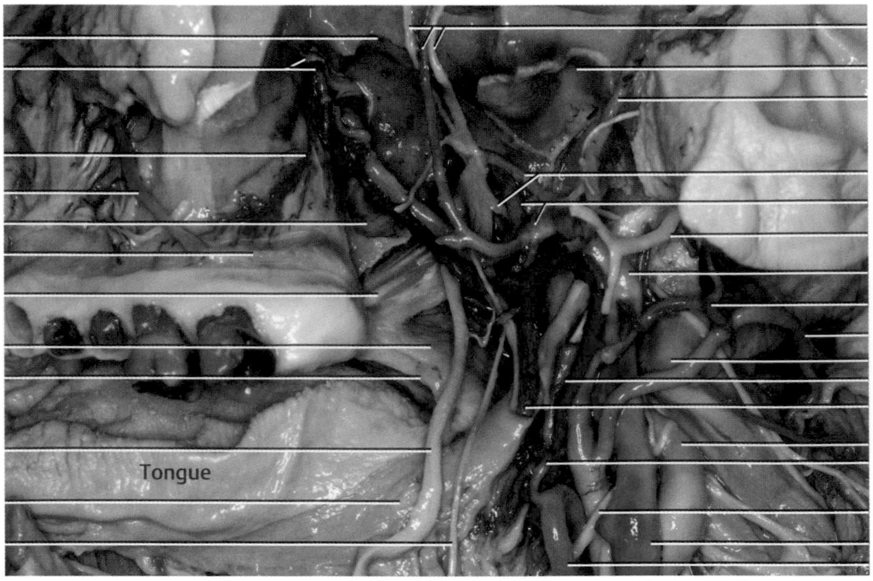

Fig. 10.8. Infratemporal fossa. The medial pterygoid muscle and the mandible have been removed.

The tensor veli palatini muscle pulls the soft palate laterally. When this muscle and the levator veli palatini muscle act together, the palatine aponeurosis becomes taut and horizontal and provides a platform upon which other palatini muscle may act to change the position of the soft palate (see **Fig. 8.6**).

The facial artery gives off the ascending palatine artery, the tonsillar artery, branches to the submandibular gland, and the submental artery in the neck.

The pterygomandibular raphe is a ligamentous band between the superior pharyngeal constrictor muscle and the middle portion of the buccinator muscle. It attaches to the pterygoid hamulus superiorly and to the posterior end of the mylohyoid line of the mandible.

The superior pharyngeal constrictor muscle originates mainly from the posterior border of the pterygomandibular raphe. This raphe provides the site of origin for both the superior constrictor and buccinator muscles. This muscle constricts the upper part of the pharynx, and it is innervated from the accessory nerve.

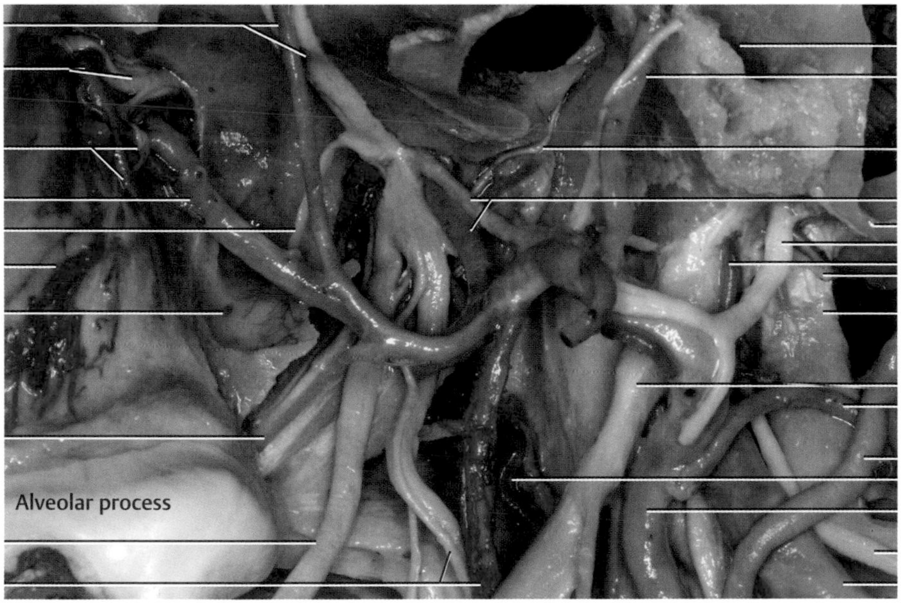

Deep temporal a., n., Masseteric n.
Infraorbital a., n.
Posterior superior alveolar a., n.
Maxillary a.
Buccal n.
Deep facial v.
Lateral pterygoid plate
Tensor veli palatini m.
Alveolar process
Lingual n.
Inferior alveolar n., a. v.

External acoustic meatus
Superficial temporal a.
Chorda tympani n. (petrotympanic fissure) (Spine of sphenoid bone has been removed)
Auriculotemporal n., Middle meningeal a.
Mastoid tip
Facial n.
Stylomastoid a.
Br. to digastric m.
Rectus capitis lateralis m.
Styloid process
Posterior auricular a.
Occipital a.
Ascending palatine a.
External carotid a.
Accessory n.
Internal jugular v.

Fig. 10.9. Infratemporal fossa. The mandibular fossa has been drilled.

The mandibular nerve is the largest division of the trigeminal nerve and has motor and sensory fibers. The sensory fibers supply the mandibular teeth, the anterior two-thirds of the tongue and the floor of the mouth, the skin of the lower part of the face, and parts of the temporal and auricular region. The mandibular nerve lies on the tensor veli palatini muscle after passing through the foramen ovale. After a short distance, the nerve divides into a smaller anterior trunk and a larger posterior trunk. Prior to this division, the main trunk gives off the meningeal branch and the nerve to the medial pterygoid muscle.

The anterior trunk has four branches: the masseteric nerve, the deep temporal nerve, the nerve to the lateral pterygoid muscle, and the buccal nerve. The posterior trunk has three branches: the auriculotemporal nerve, the lingual nerve, and the inferior alveolar nerve.

The lingual nerve is essentially a sensory nerve, but following union with the chorda tympani branch of the facial nerve, it also contains parasympathetic fibers. The nerve lies on the tensor veli palatini muscle deep to the lateral pterygoid muscle. Then the chorda tympani nerve, which has entered the infratemporal fossa via the petrotympanic fissure, joins the posterior surface of the lingual nerve.

The tensor veli palatini muscle lies lateral to the Eustachian tube. It runs downward toward the pterygoid hamulus at the inferior border of the medial pterygoid plate, and its tendon inserts in the soft palate.

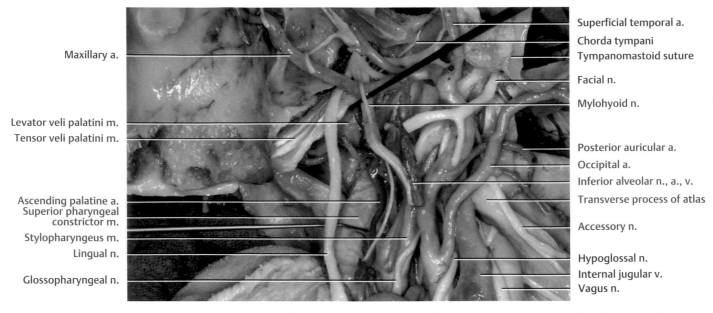

Maxillary a.

Levator veli palatini m.
Tensor veli palatini m.

Ascending palatine a.
Superior pharyngeal
constrictor m.
Stylopharyngeus m.
Lingual n.

Glossopharyngeal n.

Superficial temporal a.
Chorda tympani
Tympanomastoid suture

Facial n.

Mylohyoid n.

Posterior auricular a.
Occipital a.
Inferior alveolar n., a., v.
Transverse process of atlas

Accessory n.

Hypoglossal n.
Internal jugular v.
Vagus n.

Fig. 10.10. Infratemporal fossa. The tensor veli palatini muscle has been lifted to show the levator veli palatini muscle.

The levator veli palatini muscle is medial and slightly posterior to the tensor veli palatini muscle. It spreads to attach widely to the soft palate. This muscle forms a U-shaped muscular sling. When the palatine aponeurosis is stiffened by the tensor muscles, contraction of the levator muscles produces an upward and backward movement of the soft palate. This muscle is innervated by the accessory nerve via the pharyngeal plexus.

The ascending palatine artery arises close to the origin of the facial artery and passes up between the styloglossus and stylopharyngeus to the side of the pharynx along which it continues between the superior pharyngeal constrictor muscle and the medial pterygoid muscle to near the base of the skull.

The stylopharyngeus muscle elevates the pharynx and larynx, and it is innervated from the glossopharyngeal nerve.

The styloglossus muscle draws up the sides of the tongue to create a trough for swallowing, and it is innervated by the hypoglossal nerve like all muscles of the tongue except the palatoglossus muscle, which is innervated by the pharyngeal plexus of vagus nerve.

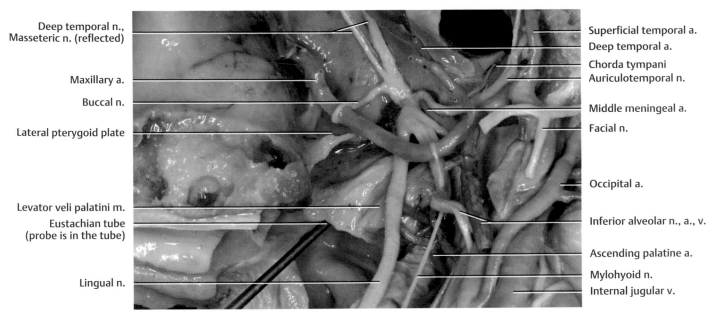

Deep temporal n.,
Masseteric n. (reflected)

Maxillary a.

Buccal n.

Lateral pterygoid plate

Levator veli palatini m.
Eustachian tube
(probe is in the tube)

Lingual n.

Superficial temporal a.
Deep temporal a.

Chorda tympani
Auriculotemporal n.

Middle meningeal a.
Facial n.

Occipital a.

Inferior alveolar n., a., v.

Ascending palatine a.

Mylohyoid n.
Internal jugular v.

Fig. 10.11. Infratemporal fossa. The tensor veli palatini muscle has been removed.

The mylohyoid nerve, which is given off from the inferior alveolar nerve just before the mandibular foramen, has motor and sensory components. It supplies the mylohyoid muscle and the anterior belly of digastric muscle. It also supplies the skin of the submental region (see **Fig. 11.4**).

The Eustachian tube is also called the auditory tube. It links the lateral wall of the nasopharynx to the anterior wall of the tympanic cavity. The Eustachian tube runs anteriorly and inferiorly from the middle ear to the nasopharynx. It has a bony part in the petrous bone and a cartilaginous part that lies in the infratemporal fossa. The cartilaginous part gives attachment to the tensor veli palatini muscle, the levator veli palatini muscle, and the salpingopharyngeus muscle. The tensor veli palatini intervenes between the tube and the mandibular nerve, the otic ganglion, the chorda tympani nerve, and the middle meningeal artery. The functions of the Eustachian tube are pressure equalization and mucus drainage. Under normal circumstances, the human Eustachian tube is closed, but it can open to let a small amount of air through to prevent damage by equalizing pressure between the middle ear and the atmosphere. The Eustachian tube drains mucus from the middle ear.

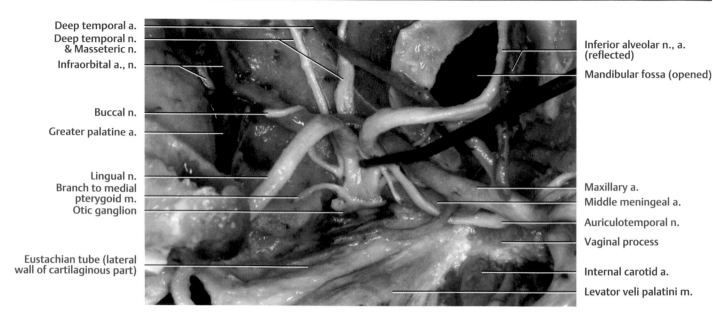

Deep temporal a.
Deep temporal n. & Masseteric n.
Infraorbital a., n.

Buccal n.
Greater palatine a.

Lingual n.
Branch to medial pterygoid m.
Otic ganglion

Eustachian tube (lateral wall of cartilaginous part)

Inferior alveolar n., a. (reflected)
Mandibular fossa (opened)

Maxillary a.
Middle meningeal a.
Auriculotemporal n.
Vaginal process

Internal carotid a.
Levator veli palatini m.

Fig. 10.12. Infratemporal fossa. The mandibular nerve has been lifted to show the otic ganglion.

The otic ganglion is a parasympathetic ganglion, which lies on the medial surface of the main trunk of the mandibular nerve immediately below the foramen ovale. It is concerned primarily with supplying the parotid gland. The parasympathetic, sympathetic, and sensory components reach the parotid gland by way of the auriculotemporal nerve. The preganglionic parasympathetic fibers originate from the inferior salivatory nucleus in the brain stem. The fibers pass out in the glossopharyngeal nerve, appearing as the lessor petrosal nerve from the tympanic plexus in the middle ear cavity. Its sympathetic postganglionic fibers consists of a filament from the plexus surrounding the middle meningeal artery.

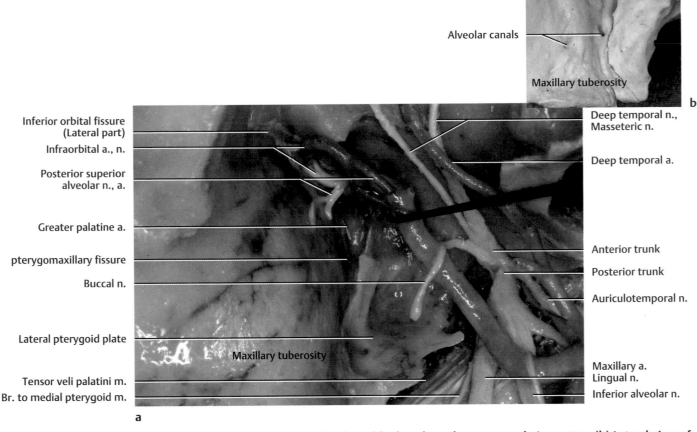

Fig. 10.13a,b. Infratemporal fossa. (a) The maxillary artery has been lifted to show the greater palatine artery. (b) Lateral view of the skull with the maxillary tuberosity highlighted.

The posterior superior alveolar nerve arises from the maxillary nerve in the pterygopalatine fossa. It descends onto the posterior wall of the maxilla and divides into dental and gingival branches. The dental branches and vessels enter the maxilla and run in the posterior alveolar canals (**Fig. 10.13b**) above the roots of the molar teeth. The three superior alveolar nerves (anterior, middle and posterior superior alveolar) form a plexus just above the roots of the maxillary teeth.

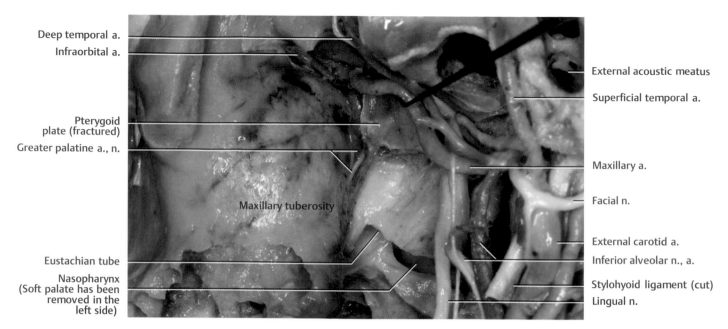

Deep temporal a.
Infraorbital a.

External acoustic meatus

Superficial temporal a.

Pterygoid
plate (fractured)

Greater palatine a., n.

Maxillary a.

Facial n.

Maxillary tuberosity

External carotid a.

Eustachian tube

Inferior alveolar n., a.

Nasopharynx
(Soft palate has been
removed in the
left side)

Stylohyoid ligament (cut)

Lingual n.

Fig. 10.14. Infratemporal fossa. The pterygoid plate has been fractured.

The pterygopalatine fossa communicates with the infratemporal fossa through the pterygomaxillary fissure. At the base of the pterygopalatine fossa, the greater and lesser palatine nerves, which arise from the pterygopalatine ganglion together with accompanying vessels (greater and lesser palatine arteries), pass into the hard palate to emerge at the greater and lesser palatine foramina (see **Fig. 8.5**).

The pterygomaxillary fissure transmits the maxillary artery from the infratemporal fossa. The fissure continues above with the posterior end of the inferior orbital fissure in the floor of the orbit.

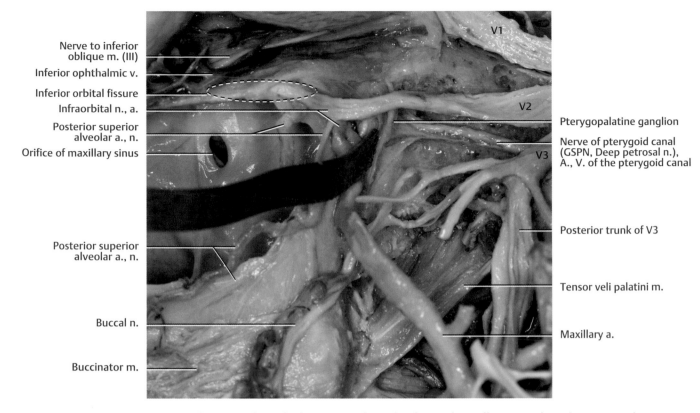

Nerve to inferior
oblique m. (III)

Inferior ophthalmic v.

Inferior orbital fissure

Infraorbital n., a.

Posterior superior
alveolar a., n.

Orifice of maxillary sinus

Posterior superior
alveolar a., n.

Buccal n.

Buccinator m.

V1

V2

V3

Pterygopalatine ganglion

Nerve of pterygoid canal
(GSPN, Deep petrosal n.),
A., V. of the pterygoid canal

Posterior trunk of V3

Tensor veli palatini m.

Maxillary a.

Fig. 10.15. The nerve of pterygoid canal. The pterygoid canal, orbit, and maxillary sinus have been opened.

The pterygoid canal (also known as the vidian canal) is a passage in the skull leading from just anterior to the foramen lacerum in the middle cranial fossa to the pterygopalatine fossa. The greater petrosal nerve (preganglionic parasympathetic), the deep petrosal nerve (postganglionic sympathetic), and accompanying vessels (artery and vein of the pterygoid canal), which originate from the pterygopalatine segment of the maxillary artery, enter the pterygoid canal. On leaving the pterygoid canal, the nerves emerge into the pterygopalatine fossa and join the pterygopalatine ganglion. From the superior cervical ganglion, sympathetic fibers pass to the internal carotid plexus and appear as the deep petrosal nerve. The deep petrosal nerve innervates the blood vessels of the lacrimal gland. The fibers do not synapse at the ganglion and pass to the lacrimal gland along the same course as the parasympathetic innervation.

The buccal nerve courses between the two heads of the lateral pterygoid muscle (see **Fig. 10.2**, **Fig. 10.3**, and **Fig. 10.4**) underneath the tendon of the temporalis muscle and then under the masseter muscle to connect with the zygomaticobuccal branches of the facial nerve on the surface of the buccinator muscle (see **Fig. 11.6**).

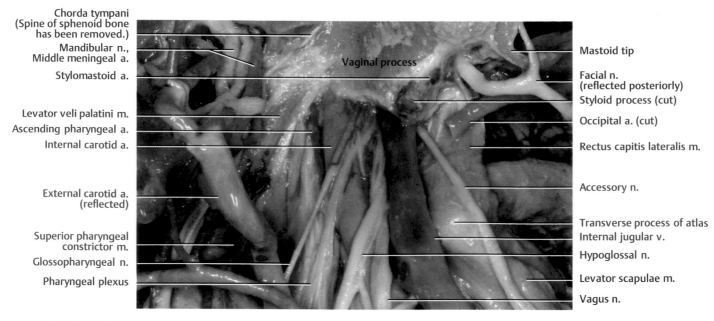

Chorda tympani
(Spine of sphenoid bone
has been removed.)
Mandibular n.,
Middle meningeal a.

Stylomastoid a.

Levator veli palatini m.
Ascending pharyngeal a.
Internal carotid a.

External carotid a.
(reflected)

Superior pharyngeal
constrictor m.
Glossopharyngeal n.

Pharyngeal plexus

Vaginal process

Mastoid tip

Facial n.
(reflected posteriorly)
Styloid process (cut)

Occipital a. (cut)

Rectus capitis lateralis m.

Accessory n.

Transverse process of atlas
Internal jugular v.

Hypoglossal n.

Levator scapulae m.

Vagus n.

Fig. 10.16. Structures adjacent to the facial nerve trunk. The styloid process has been cut and the facial nerve has been reflected laterally.

The stylomastoid artery, which generally originates from the posterior auricular artery or the occipital artery, supplies the facial nerve trunk and enters into the skull, close to the facial nerve, through the stylomastoid foramen.

The hypoglossal nerve passes between the internal jugular vein and the internal carotid artery to the level of the transverse process of the atlas, where it turns abruptly forward along the lateral surface of the internal carotid artery toward the tongue, leaving only the ansa cervicalis to descend with the major vessels. It then runs anteriorly between the internal and external carotid arteries and onto the stylopharyngeus muscle. It passes below the submandibular gland onto the hyoglossus muscle to be distributed to the muscle of the tongue (see **Fig. 12.2**). The hypoglossal nerve is a source of axons for facial reinnervation when the proximal facial nerve stump is not available but the distal facial nerve and facial musculature are present and functional.

Through the jugular foramen, the accessory nerve descends obliquely, crosses the internal jugular vein (usually on its lateral surface), and runs then backward and downward to reach the upper part of the sternocleidomastoid muscle (see **Fig. 12.3**). Approximately 30% of nerves descend along the medial, rather than the lateral, surface of the internal jugular vein. The spinal accessory nerve provides motor innervation to two muscles of the neck: the sternocleidomastoid and the trapezius.

The glossopharyngeal nerve leaves the skull through the jugular foramen and passes between the internal jugular vein and the internal carotid artery. The glossopharyngeal nerve is mostly sensory, with only one motor component. Glossopharyngeal nerve gets pain, temperature, and touch from the tongue, ear, insides of the throat, and so on. It gets taste from the back one-third of the tongue.

The pharyngeal plexus, with fibers from CN IX, CN X, and cranial part of CN XI, innervates all the muscles of the pharynx except the stylopharyngeus muscle, which is innervated by CN IX. The plexus provides sensory innervation of the oropharynx and laryngopharynx.

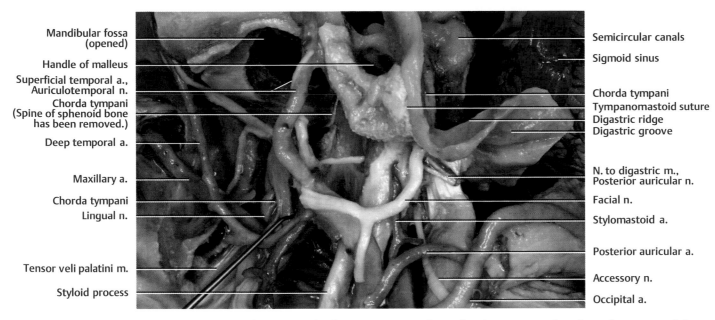

Mandibular fossa (opened)

Handle of malleus

Superficial temporal a., Auriculotemporal n.

Chorda tympani (Spine of sphenoid bone has been removed.)

Deep temporal a.

Maxillary a.

Chorda tympani

Lingual n.

Tensor veli palatini m.

Styloid process

Semicircular canals

Sigmoid sinus

Chorda tympani
Tympanomastoid suture
Digastric ridge
Digastric groove

N. to digastric m., Posterior auricular n.

Facial n.

Stylomastoid a.

Posterior auricular a.

Accessory n.

Occipital a.

Fig. 10.17. Structures adjacent to the facial nerve trunk. The tympanic membrane has been removed to show the course of the chorda tympani.

The chorda tympani is given off just before the stylomastoid foramen from the mastoid segment of the facial nerve. This is the branch from the nervus intermedius. It contains parasympathetic fibers going to the submandibular ganglion and taste fibers from the anterior two-thirds of the tongue. The nerve initially runs within its own canal before entering the tympanic cavity. It travels through the middle ear, where it runs from posterior to anterior across the tympanic membrane. It passes between the malleus and the incus on the medial surface of the neck of the malleus. The nerve continues through the petrotympanic fissure, after which it emerges from the skull into the infratemporal fossa. It soon combines with the lingual nerve at the infratemporal fossa.

The digastric ridge, which is a ridge of bone, corresponds to the digastric groove and marks the location of the facial canal just anterior to it.

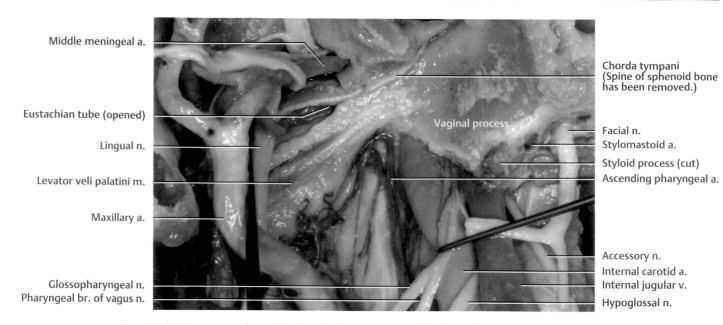

Middle meningeal a.

Chorda tympani
(Spine of sphenoid bone
has been removed.)

Eustachian tube (opened)

Vaginal process

Facial n.

Lingual n.

Stylomastoid a.

Styloid process (cut)

Levator veli palatini m.

Ascending pharyngeal a.

Maxillary a.

Accessory n.

Internal carotid a.

Glossopharyngeal n.

Internal jugular v.

Pharyngeal br. of vagus n.

Hypoglossal n.

Fig. 10.18. Structures adjacent to the facial nerve trunk. The Eustachian tube has been opened.

The ascending pharyngeal artery is the smallest branch of the external carotid artery. It arises from the posterior surface of the external carotid artery, passing vertically upward to the pharynx. It terminates near the base of the skull. The meningeal branches from the ascending pharyngeal artery enter through the foramen lacerum and the hypoglossal canal.

The middle cranial fossa is innervated by the meningeal branch of the mandibular division of the trigeminal nerve. It enters the cranial cavity through the foramen spinosum.

The middle meningeal artery is the main source of blood to the meninges and to the bones of the vault of the skull. It ascends between the two roots of the auriculotemporal nerve and leaves the infratemporal fossa through the foramen spinosum.

Both the jugular foramen and carotid canal are situated behind the vaginal process, which encloses the root of the styloid process and forms the posterior wall of the condylar fossa.

III Lower Facial and Posterolateral Neck Region

11 Lower Facial Region

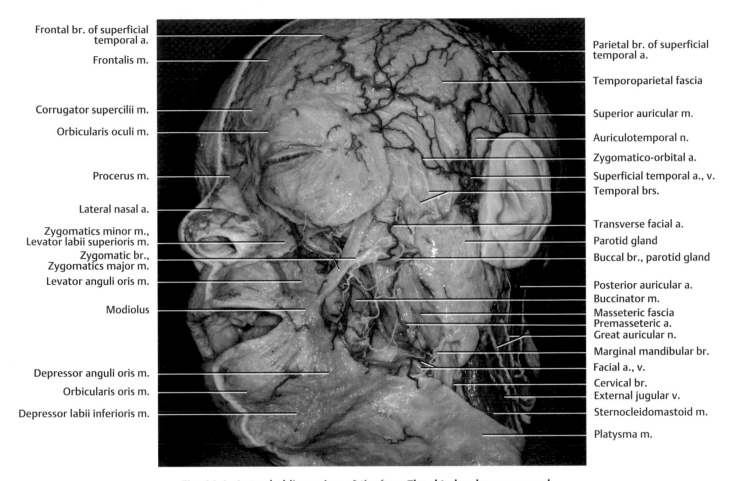

Frontal br. of superficial temporal a.

Frontalis m.

Corrugator supercilii m.

Orbicularis oculi m.

Procerus m.

Lateral nasal a.

Zygomatics minor m., Levator labii superioris m.

Zygomatic br., Zygomatics major m.

Levator anguli oris m.

Modiolus

Depressor anguli oris m.

Orbicularis oris m.

Depressor labii inferioris m.

Parietal br. of superficial temporal a.

Temporoparietal fascia

Superior auricular m.

Auriculotemporal n.

Zygomatico-orbital a.

Superficial temporal a., v.
Temporal brs.

Transverse facial a.

Parotid gland

Buccal br., parotid gland

Posterior auricular a.

Buccinator m.

Masseteric fascia
Premasseteric a.
Great auricular n.

Marginal mandibular br.

Facial a., v.

Cervical br.

External jugular v.

Sternocleidomastoid m.

Platysma m.

Fig. 11.1. Lateral oblique view of the face. The skin has been removed.

The modiolus is a nodular region at the corner of the mouth where several mimetic muscles converge and interlace. It is contributed by the orbicularis oris, buccinator, levator anguli oris, depressor anguli oris, zygomatics major, and risorius muscles.

The depressor labii inferioris muscle is partly covered by the anterior fibers of the depressor anguli oris muscle.

The levator anguli oris, the buccinator, and the mentalis muscles are deep-seated muscles that are innervated on their superficial surface by the facial nerve branches.

The facial vein begins as the angular vein at the medial corner of the eye. The angular vein is formed by the confluence of the supraorbital and supratrochlear veins. The facial vein passes downward behind the facial artery independently to the inferior border of the mandible.

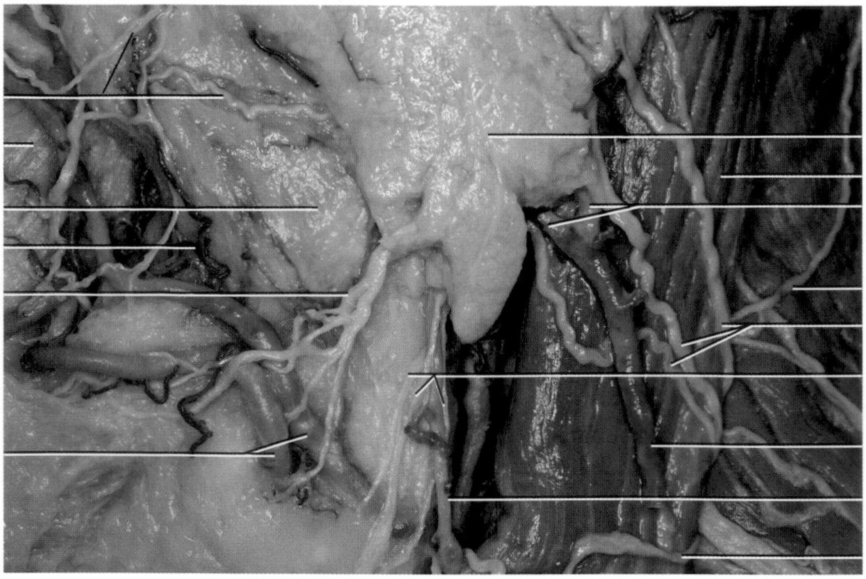

Buccal brs. (masseteric fascia is opened)
Buccinator m.
Masseteric fascia
Premasseteric artery
Marginal mandibular br.
Facial a., v.

Tail of parotid gland
Sternocleidomastoid m.
Posterior auricular v., posterior br. of retromandibular v.
Lesser occipital n.
Great auricular n.
Cervical brs.
External jugular v.
Anterior br. of retromandibular v.
Transverse cervical n.

Fig. 11.2. The lower facial region. Close up view of the parotid tail and mandibular angle.

The marginal mandibular branches of the facial nerve emerge from the lower border of the parotid gland, and the branch runs near the inferior border of the mandible. Initially, it may pass into the neck below the angle of the mandible, but after crossing the facial artery it usually comes up above the lower border of the mandible to the face. It innervates the depressor anguli oris, the depressor labii inferioris, the mentalis, and the lower orbicularis oris muscles.

The cervical branch passes downward from the lower border of the parotid gland to supply the platysma muscle in the neck. Some of the its branches frequently innervate the depressor labii inferioris and the depressor anguli oris muscles.

One of the buccal branches runs beneath the masseteric fascia in this figure. However, most of the marginal mandibular branches generally run on the fascia.

At the inferior border of the mandible near the anterior edge of the masseter muscle, the facial artery and the vein course closely.

The premasseteric artery arises at the lower border of the mandible from the facial artery and ascends along the anterior edge of the masseter muscle.

The great auricular nerve perforates the deep cervical fascia and ascends upon the sternocleidomastoid muscle beneath the platysma to the parotid gland, where it divides into an anterior and a posterior branch. It provides sensory innervation for the skin over the parotid gland and the mastoid process, as well as both surfaces of the caudal region of the auricle.

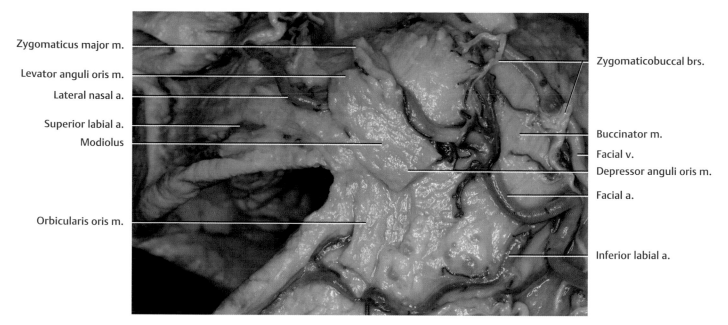

Zygomaticus major m.

Levator anguli oris m.

Lateral nasal a.

Superior labial a.

Modiolus

Orbicularis oris m.

Zygomaticobuccal brs.

Buccinator m.

Facial v.

Depressor anguli oris m.

Facial a.

Inferior labial a.

Fig. 11.3. The lower facial region. Close up view of the oral commissure.

The modiolus may be fixed by the action of some of the muscles to provide a base for the action of other muscles.

The orbicularis oris muscle is a complex of muscles in the lips that encircle the mouth. This muscle closes the mouth and puckers the lips when it contracts. It is innervated by the zygomaticobuccal branch and the marginal mandibular branch.

The facial artery passes upward and forward from the mandible and lies deep to the zygomaticus major muscle and superficial to the buccinator muscle. It lies either superficial or deep to the levator anguli oris muscle and levator labii superioris muscle. The branches of the facial artery on the face are the inferior labial and superior labial. It terminates as lateral nasal arteries or the angular artery. The former two branches are situated deep to the orbicularis oris muscle.

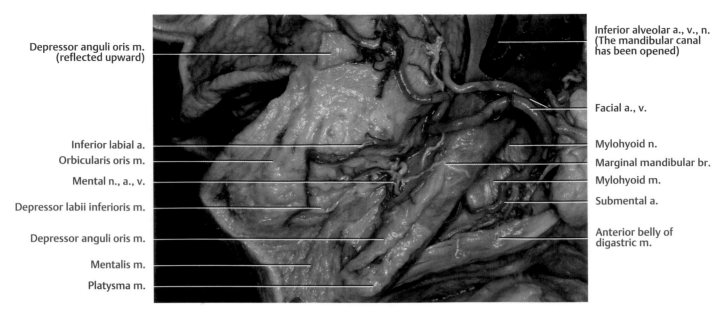

Depressor anguli oris m.
(reflected upward)

Inferior labial a.

Orbicularis oris m.

Mental n., a., v.

Depressor labii inferioris m.

Depressor anguli oris m.

Mentalis m.

Platysma m.

Inferior alveolar a., v., n.
(The mandibular canal
has been opened)

Facial a., v.

Mylohyoid n.

Marginal mandibular br.

Mylohyoid m.

Submental a.

Anterior belly of
digastric m.

Fig. 11.4. The lower facial region. The platysma and depressor anguli oris muscles have been removed to leave their attachments.

The mentalis muscle is in the deepest layer among the mimetic muscles. It originates from the incisive fossa of the mandible. Its fibers descend to insert into the skin of the chin. This muscle raises and protrudes the lower lip.

The depressor labii inferioris muscle arises from the mandible just in front of the mental foramen. The fibers pass upward and medially to converge with the orbicularis oris muscle in the lower lip. This muscle depresses the lower lip and draws it laterally.

The depressor anguli oris muscle arises from an extensive area around the external oblique line of the mandible. Its fibers pass upward to the corner of the mouth. This muscle depresses the corner of the mouth.

The platysma muscle is a flat muscle which inserts into the subcutaneous tissues of the subclavicular and acromial regions inferiorly and then inserts into the chin at the commissures of the mouth and in the anterior one-third of the oblique line of the mandible. This muscle is a depressor of the lower lip innervated by the cervical branch of the facial nerve.

The digastric muscle stretches between the mastoid process of the cranium to the mandible. Part of the way between, it becomes a tendon that passes through a tendinous pulley attached to the hyoid bone. The anterior belly of the digastric muscle arises from a depression on the inner side of the lower border of the mandible called the digastric fossa, which is close to the symphysis, and passes downward and backward.

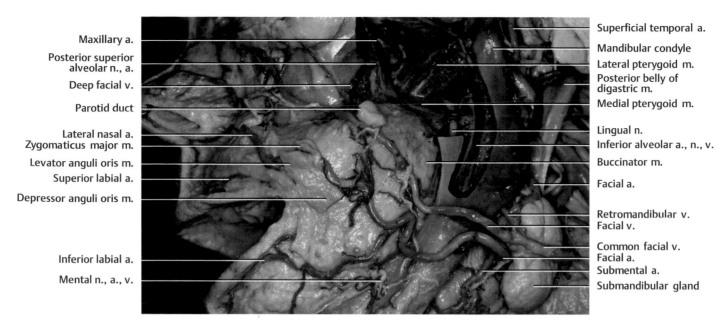

Maxillary a.
Posterior superior alveolar n., a.
Deep facial v.
Parotid duct
Lateral nasal a.
Zygomaticus major m.
Levator anguli oris m.
Superior labial a.
Depressor anguli oris m.
Inferior labial a.
Mental n., a., v.

Superficial temporal a.
Mandibular condyle
Lateral pterygoid m.
Posterior belly of digastric m.
Medial pterygoid m.
Lingual n.
Inferior alveolar a., n., v.
Buccinator m.
Facial a.
Retromandibular v.
Facial v.
Common facial v.
Facial a.
Submental a.
Submandibular gland

Fig. 11.5. The lower facial region. The mandibular canal has been opened.

The buccinator muscle is in the deepest layer among the mimetic muscles, and it functions principally during mastication. An important relationship is with the parotid duct, which pierces the muscle opposite the maxillary third molar and then runs forward to open into the oral cavity opposite the maxillary second molar. This muscle has two main origins. First, it arises from the anterior margin of the pterygomandibular raphe. Second, it is attached to the alveolar margins of the maxilla and mandible in the region of the molar teeth. The fibers eventually run into the orbicularis oris muscle.

The inferior alveolar nerve arises from the mandibular nerve and emerges from beneath the lateral pterygoid muscle. Then, it gives off a mylohyoid branch which has motor and sensory components. It next enters the mandible with the vessels via the mandibular foramen. While in the mandibular canal within the mandible, the main trunk of the inferior alveolar nerve divides near the premolars into mental and incisive nerves. The mental nerve and vessels run for a short distance in a mental canal before leaving the body of the mandible at the mental foramen to emerge onto the face. It supplies the skin and mucosa of the lower lip and the labial gingivae of the mandibular anterior teeth. The mental nerve has communication with the marginal mandibular branch of the facial nerve. The mental artery arises from the mandibular segment of the maxillary artery as a terminal branch of the inferior alveolar artery.

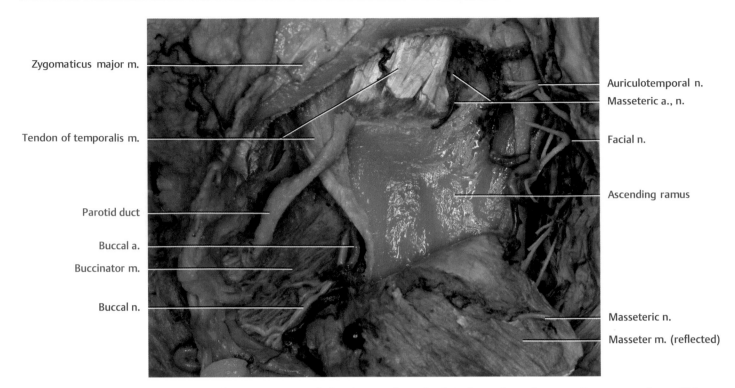

Zygomaticus major m.

Tendon of temporalis m.

Parotid duct

Buccal a.

Buccinator m.

Buccal n.

Auriculotemporal n.

Masseteric a., n.

Facial n.

Ascending ramus

Masseteric n.

Masseter m. (reflected)

Fig. 11.6. The lower facial region. The masseter muscle has been reflected inferiorly to show the ascending ramus of mandible.

The buccal nerve runs into the upper part of the retromolar fossa at the anterior border of the ramus of the mandible. The buccal nerve divides into several branches within the buccinator muscle. It innervates both the mucosa and the skin of the cheek and buccal gingivae of the mandibular cheek teeth. The buccal nerve has communication with zygomaticobuccal branches of the facial nerve.

The buccal artery is a branch of the pterygoid segment of the maxillary artery. It emerges onto the face from the infratemporal fossa and crosses the buccinator muscle to supply the cheek. The masseteric artery is also a branch of the pterygoid segment of the maxillary artery and courses close to the same nerve anteroinferiorly in the masseter muscle.

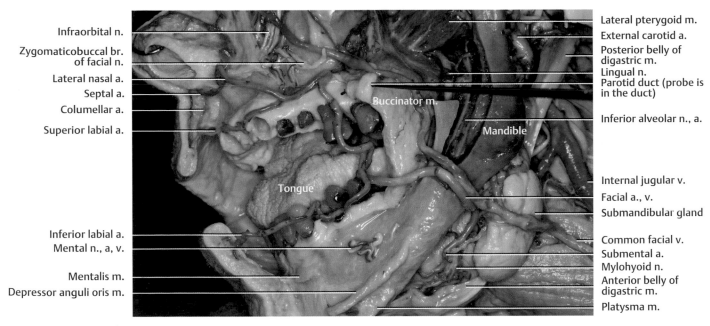

Infraorbital n.
Zygomaticobuccal br. of facial n.
Lateral nasal a.
Septal a.
Columellar a.
Superior labial a.
Buccinator m.
Tongue
Inferior labial a.
Mental n., a., v.
Mentalis m.
Depressor anguli oris m.

Lateral pterygoid m.
External carotid a.
Posterior belly of digastric m.
Lingual n.
Parotid duct (probe is in the duct)
Inferior alveolar n., a.
Mandible
Internal jugular v.
Facial a., v.
Submandibular gland
Common facial v.
Submental a.
Mylohyoid n.
Anterior belly of digastric m.
Platysma m.

Fig. 11.7. The lower facial region. The upper and lower lip have been removed to leave the facial artery.

The facial artery usually lies anterior to the facial vein throughout its course and courses close to the vein on the mandible.

The superior labial artery is larger and more egregious than the inferior labial artery. It courses along the edge of the upper lip, lying between the mucous membrane and the orbicularis oris muscle, and it anastomoses with the artery of the opposite side. It supplies the upper lip and gives off in its course two branches that ascend to the nose: a septal branch ramifies on the nasal septum and a columellar branch supplies the columella of the nose.

The inferior labial artery arises near the angle of the mouth. It passes upward and forward beneath the depressor anguli oris muscle and, penetrating the orbicularis oris muscle, runs in a tortuous course along the edge of the lower lip between this muscle and the mucous membrane. It supplies the labial glands, the mucous membrane, and the muscles of the lower lip, and it anastomoses with the artery of the opposite side

The submental artery is a branch of the facial artery, given off just as that vessel leaves the submandibular gland. It runs forward upon the mylohyoid, just below the body of the mandible and beneath the digastric muscle. It supplies the surrounding muscles and also a territory of skin in the submental area.

12 Oral Floor and Upper Neck Region

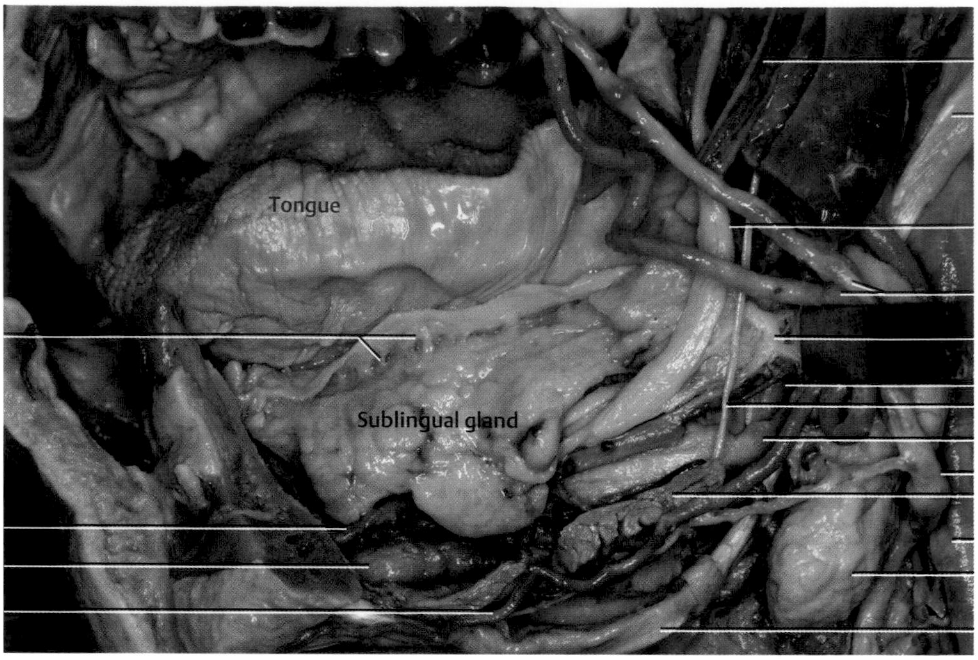

Inferior alveolar n., a., v.

Posterior belly of digastric m.

Lingual n.

Facial a., v.

Submandibular ganglion

Hyoglossus m.
Mylohyoid n.
Hypoglossal n.
Common facial v.
Mylohyoid m.

Internal jugular v.

Submandibular Gland

Anterior belly of digastric m.

Tongue

Ducts of sublingual gland

Sublingual gland

Sublingual a.

Geniohyoid m.

Submental a.

Fig. 12.1. The oral floor from the side. Part of the mandible has been removed.

The submandibular ganglion is parasympathetic ganglion that is found in the floor of the mouth on the superficial surface of the hyoglossus muscle. It lies between the lingual nerve and the deep part of the submandibular gland. It is suspended by two roots from the lingual nerve. The submandibular ganglion is responsible for innervation of the submandibular gland and sublingual gland. Preganglionic parasympathetic fibers originate from the superior salivary nucleus in the brain stem. The fibers pass with the nervus intermedius of the facial nerve into the internal acoustic meatus and exit the skull with the chorda tympani at the petrotympanic fissure. The chorda tympani nerve joins the lingual nerve.

The inferior alveolar nerve branches off the mylohyoid nerve before entering the mandibular canal. The mylohyoid nerve courses inferiorly and anteriorly in the mylohyoid groove beneath the mylohyoid line (see **Fig. 3.7**). It supplies the mylohyoid muscle and the anterior belly of digastric muscle. It also supplies the skin of the submental region.

The lingual nerve courses toward the floor of the mouth from the infratemporal fossa. It supplies the mucosa covering the anterior two-thirds of the dorsum of the tongue, the ventral surface of the tongue, the floor of the mouth, and the lingual gingivae of the mandibular teeth. The rest of the posterior part of the tongue are innervated by the glossopharyngeal nerve.

The mylohyoid muscle arises from the mylohyoid line on the medial surface of the body of the mandible. Its fibers interdigitate with the contralateral fibers to form a medial raphe. This raphe is attached above to the mandible and below to the hyoid bone. The muscle raises the floor of the mouth during the first stages of swallowing. It also helps to depress the mandible when hyoid bone is fixed. Conversely, it aids in elevation of the hyoid bone.

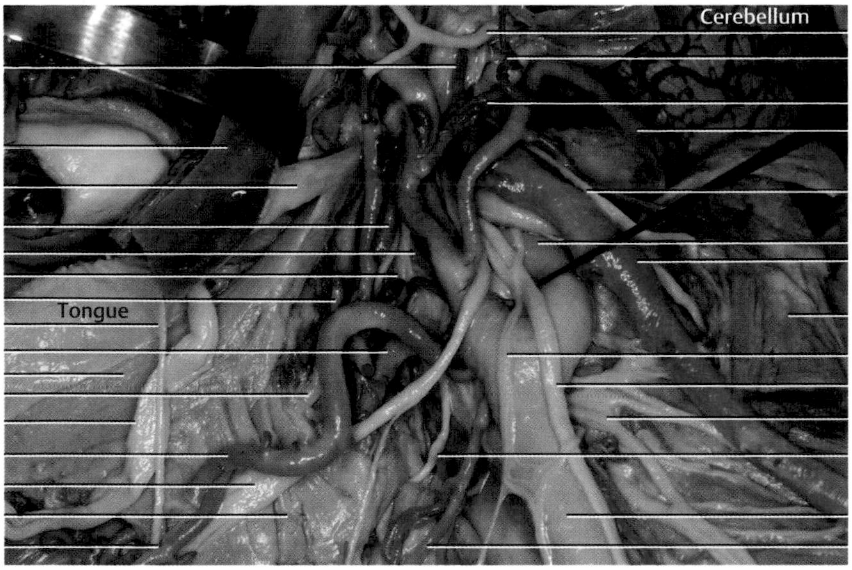

Fig. 12.2. The upper neck region. The branches of the external carotid artery.

The common carotid artery divides at the upper border of the thyroid cartilage, which is generally on a level with the upper border of the fourth cervical vertebra. At its origin, the external carotid artery is actually anteromedial to the internal carotid artery. The external carotid artery ascends anteriorly to the internal carotid artery through the parotid gland, deep to the retromandibular vein. Proximal to its terminal bifurcation into the maxillary and the superficial temporal arteries, it gives rise to six branches: the superior thyroid artery, the ascending pharyngeal artery, the lingual artery, the facial artery, the occipital artery, and the posterior auricular artery.

The superior thyroid artery is the first branch of the external carotid artery. It arises at the level of the greater horn of the hyoid bone and supplies the thyroid, the sternocleidomastoid muscle, and the larynx.

The ascending pharyngeal artery is the smallest branch of the external carotid artery. It is a long, slender vessel, deeply seated in the neck beneath the other branches of the external carotid and under the stylopharyngeus muscle. It arises from the posterior surface of the external carotid artery and passes vertically upward between the internal carotid and the side of the pharynx to under the surface of the base of the skull, lying on the longus capitis muscle.

The lingual artery arises from the external carotid artery just above the superior thyroid artery and passes beneath the hyoglossus muscle to enter the tongue. Its branches are the infrahyoid artery and the sublingual artery, with the deep lingual artery as its terminal branch.

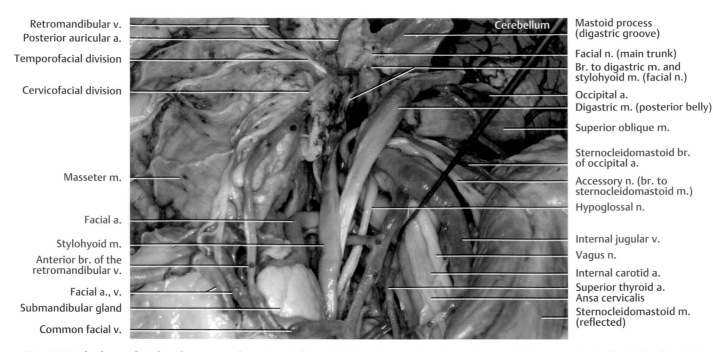

Retromandibular v.
Posterior auricular a.

Temporofacial division

Cervicofacial division

Masseter m.

Facial a.

Stylohyoid m.

Anterior br. of the
retromandibular v.

Facial a., v.

Submandibular gland

Common facial v.

Cerebellum

Mastoid process
(digastric groove)

Facial n. (main trunk)
Br. to digastric m. and
stylohyoid m. (facial n.)

Occipital a.
Digastric m. (posterior belly)

Superior oblique m.

Sternocleidomastoid br.
of occipital a.

Accessory n. (br. to
sternocleidomastoid m.)

Hypoglossal n.

Internal jugular v.

Vagus n.

Internal carotid a.

Superior thyroid a.
Ansa cervicalis

Sternocleidomastoid m.
(reflected)

Fig. 12.3. The lower facial and upper neck region. Suboccipital craniotomy has been done and the posterior belly of the digastric muscle has been detached from the digastric groove.

The branches of the facial nerve to the posterior belly of the digastric and stylohyoid muscles arise close to the stylomastoid foramen. The stylohyoid muscle is inserted into the body of the hyoid bone. When it contracts, it elevates the hyoid. This action is primarily brought about during swallowing. The muscle is perforated near its insertion by the intermediate tendon of the digastric muscle.

The ansa cervicalis is a loop of nerves that are part of the cervical plexus. The upper root of the ansa cervicalis is derived from the ventral ramus of the first cervical nerve. This branch first appears as the hypoglossal nerve loops around the occipital artery. It passes down on the carotid sheath covering the carotid arteries and is joined by the lower root of the ansa cervicalis from the cervical plexus to form the ansa cervicalis. Branches from the ansa cervicalis innervate most of the infra-

hyoid muscle, including the sternothyroid muscle, the sternohyoid muscle, and the omohyoid muscle.

The facial artery arises from the external carotid artery immediately above the greater horn of the hyoid bone. It runs upward behind the submandibular gland deep to the stylohyoid muscle and posterior belly of digastric muscle. Above the stylohyoid muscle, it turns downward and forward between the lateral surface of the submandibular gland and the medial pterygoid muscle to reach the lower border of the mandible.

The vagus nerve exits through the jugular foramen and passes into the carotid sheath between the internal carotid artery and the internal jugular vein down below the head to the neck, the chest, and the abdomen, where it contributes to the innervation of the viscera.

13 Posterior Neck and Occipital Region

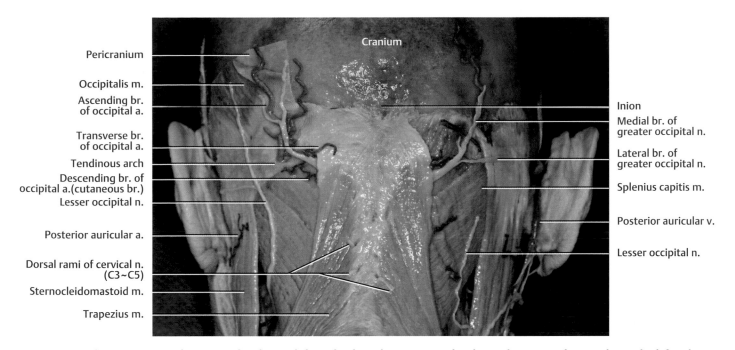

Pericranium

Occipitalis m.

Ascending br.
of occipital a.

Transverse br.
of occipital a.

Tendinous arch

Descending br. of
occipital a.(cutaneous br.)

Lesser occipital n.

Posterior auricular a.

Dorsal rami of cervical n.
(C3~C5)

Sternocleidomastoid m.

Trapezius m.

Cranium

Inion

Medial br. of
greater occipital n.

Lateral br. of
greater occipital n.

Splenius capitis m.

Posterior auricular v.

Lesser occipital n.

Fig. 13.1. The posterior neck region. The skin and the galea have been removed to leave the occipitalis muscle on the left side.

The occipitalis muscle has two muscle bellies that are separated in the midline by the aponeurosis. Each occipital belly arises from the lateral two-thirds of the supreme nuchal line of the occipital bone and from the mastoid process of the temporal bone. The muscle extends forward to become continuous with the galea aponeurotica. It is a part of the occipitofrontalis muscle, along with the frontalis muscle. It is innervated by the posterior auricular branch of the facial nerve. Its function is to move the scalp back.

The greater occipital nerve and occipital artery reach the subcutaneous tissues by passing between the attachment of the trapezius and sternocleidomastoid muscles to the superior nuchal line. The occipital artery crosses deep to the greater occipital nerve approximately 4 cm lateral to the external occipital protuberance (inion). After it pierces the deep fascia, it gives rise to three major cutaneous branches: descending, transverse, and ascending. The greater occipital nerve branches into medial and lateral branches around the superior nuchal line. It supplies the skin over the occipital part of the scalp up to the vertex of the skull.

The lesser occipital nerve has a variable origin either from the second or the second and third cervical ventral rami. The lesser occipital nerve lies at approximately 7 cm lateral to the external occipital protuberance. This nerve supplies the skin over the scalp and cranial surface of the upper part of the auricle.

The medial branches of the dorsal rami of the third, fourth, and fifth cervical nerves pierce the trapezius muscle at its paramedian position to supply skin over the back of the neck.

The trapezius muscle covers the back of the head and neck. It extends from the medial half of the superior nuchal line, the external occipital protuberance, and the spinous processes of the cervical and thoracic vertebrae and converges on the shoulder to attach to the scapula and the lateral third of the clavicle.

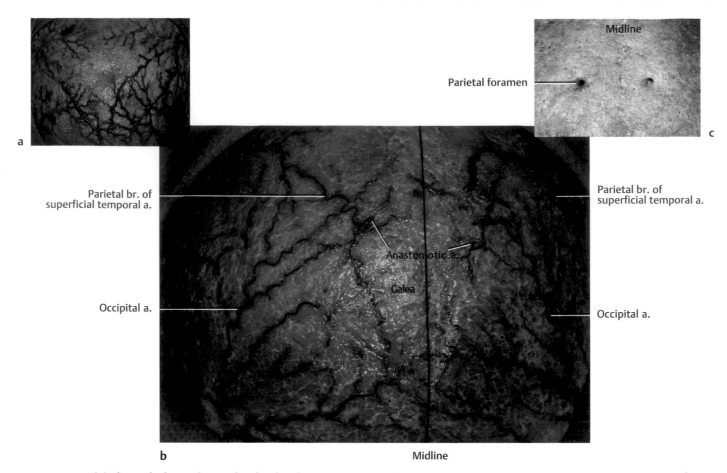

Fig. 13.2a-c. **(a) The scalp from above. The skin has been removed to show the galea. (b) The scalp from above. The scalp without pericranium has been reversed. (c) The skull from above.**

The branches from the superficial temporal, posterior auricular, occipital, supraorbital, and supratrochlear arteries freely anastomose in the scalp.

This figure shows the meningeal branch (anastomotic artery) from the occipital artery bilaterally which is passing through the parietal foramen. The well-developed anastomotic artery is found in approximately 50% of specimens, and it develops the vascular network of the galea and scalp. The rich vascular connection in the galea and scalp contributes rich vascularity to galeal and scalp flap in the head.

The parietal foramen is found in more than 60% of skulls. It may be unilateral or bilateral or duplicate on one or both sides. The vertical distance from the inion to the level of the parietal foramen is approximately 8 cm, and the distance from the midline to the foramen is within 10 mm (**Fig. 13.2c**).

The superficial temporal artery that supplies the galea does not cross the midline or anastomose with the contralateral superficial temporal artery on the galeal layer. The vein on the galea generally runs superficially on the artery except for the vertex region. The artery in the vertex region courses more superficially on the vein and anastomoses with the contralateral artery in the subcutaneous layer (**Fig. 13.2a**).

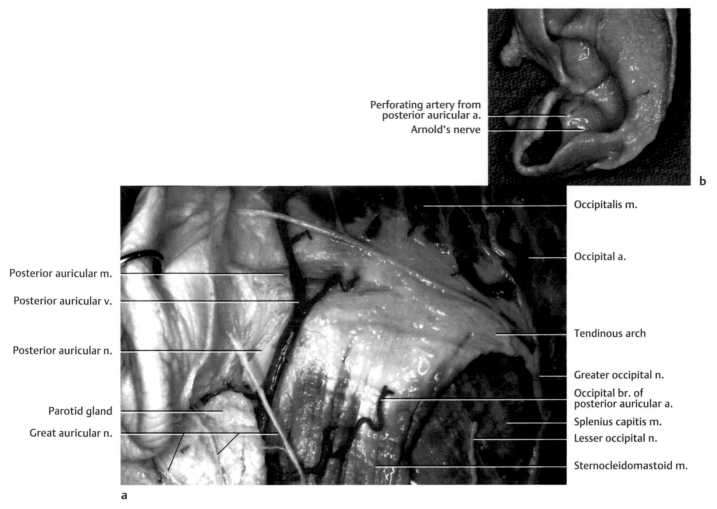

Perforating artery from posterior auricular a.

Arnold's nerve

Occipitalis m.

Occipital a.

Posterior auricular m.

Posterior auricular v.

Tendinous arch

Posterior auricular n.

Greater occipital n.

Occipital br. of posterior auricular a.

Parotid gland

Splenius capitis m.

Great auricular n.

Lesser occipital n.

Sternocleidomastoid m.

a

b

Fig. 13.3a,b. (a) The posterior neck region. (b) Lateral view of the auricular cartilage.

The posterior auricular nerve is the first extracranial branch of the facial nerve. It originates from the facial nerve close to the stylomastoid foramen and then courses posteriorly and upward on the surface of the mastoid bone. There, it is joined by a filament from the auricular branch of the vagus (see the text accompanying **Fig. 2.2**), which supplies the auricular concha as the Arnold's nerve (**Fig. 13.3b**) and communicates with the posterior branch of the great auricular, as well as the lesser occipital, nerve. It supplies the posterior auricular and occipital muscles. The posterior auricular muscle arises from the mastoid bone and inserts into cranial surface of the concha. It displaces the auricle backward.

The occipital branch of the posterior auricular artery runs back over the insertion of sternomastoid muscle to supply the skin of behind the ear. The posterior auricular vein is variable. The well-developed posterior auricular vein might be found to compensate for the underdeveloped superficial temporal vein (see **Fig. 4.2**).

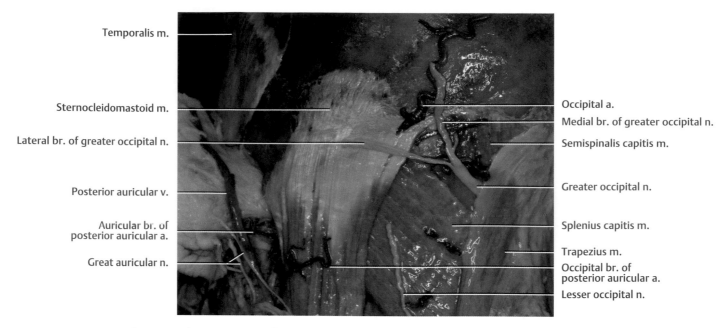

Temporalis m.

Sternocleidomastoid m.

Lateral br. of greater occipital n.

Posterior auricular v.

Auricular br. of
posterior auricular a.

Great auricular n.

Occipital a.

Medial br. of greater occipital n.

Semispinalis capitis m.

Greater occipital n.

Splenius capitis m.

Trapezius m.

Occipital br. of
posterior auricular a.

Lesser occipital n.

Fig. 13.4. The posterior neck region. The galea and occipitalis muscle have been removed.

The sternocleidomastoid muscle passes obliquely downward across the side of the neck from the lateral half of superior nuchal line and mastoid process to the upper part of the sternum and adjacent part of the clavicle. The sternocleidomastoid muscle is innervated by the accessory nerve. The function of this muscle is to rotate the head to the opposite side or obliquely rotate the head. When the muscle and nerve act together, the neck flexes and the head extends. The sternocleidomastoid branches of the occipital artery supply the cephalic end of sternocleidomastoid muscle. The spinal part of the accessory nerve supplies the sternocleidomastoid muscle and passes through or deep to it to emerge into the posterior triangle on the way to the trapezius muscle (see **Fig. 12.3**).

The sternocleidomastoid muscle divides the side of the neck into an anterior triangle and a posterior triangle. The anterior triangle is bounded posteriorly by the anterior border of the sternocleidomastoid, above by the mandible, and anteriorly by the median line of the neck; the posterior triangle is bounded in front by the posterior border of the sternocleidomastoid, below by the middle third of the clavicle, and behind by the anterior margin of the trapezius muscle.

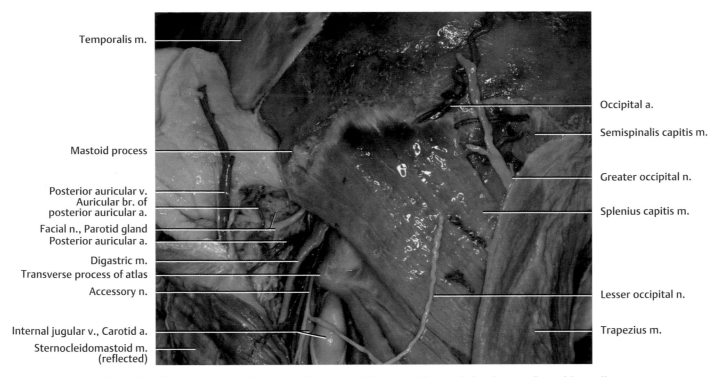

Temporalis m.

Mastoid process

Posterior auricular v.
Auricular br. of
posterior auricular a.

Facial n., Parotid gland
Posterior auricular a.

Digastric m.
Transverse process of atlas

Accessory n.

Internal jugular v., Carotid a.

Sternocleidomastoid m.
(reflected)

Occipital a.

Semispinalis capitis m.

Greater occipital n.

Splenius capitis m.

Lesser occipital n.

Trapezius m.

Fig. 13.5. The posterior neck region. The sternocleidomastoid muscle has been reflected laterally.

The posterior auricular artery is a small artery that arises from the external carotid artery above the digastric muscle and stylohyoid muscle opposite the apex of the styloid process. It ascends over the digastric muscle between the auricular cartilage and the mastoid process, pierces the deep fascia at the level of the external auditory meatus, and divides into auricular and occipital branches. The auricular branch ascends deep to posterior auricular muscle and anastomoses with the superficial temporal artery. The auricular branch has small branches which pierce the auricular cartilage to reach the external surface (see **Fig. 13.3b**).

The splenius capitis, situated deep to and partially covered by trapezius and sternocleidomastoid, extends from the bone below the lateral third of the superior nuchal line to the spinous processes of the lower cervical and upper thoracic vertebrae.

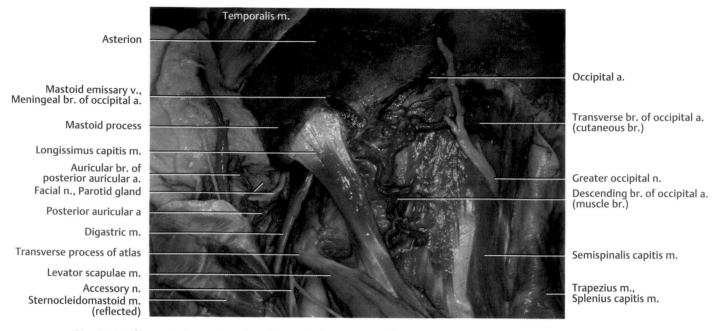

Asterion

Mastoid emissary v.,
Meningeal br. of occipital a.

Mastoid process

Longissimus capitis m.

Auricular br. of
posterior auricular a.
Facial n., Parotid gland

Posterior auricular a

Digastric m.

Transverse process of atlas

Levator scapulae m.

Accessory n.
Sternocleidomastoid m.
(reflected)

Temporalis m.

Occipital a.

Transverse br. of occipital a.
(cutaneous br.)

Greater occipital n.

Descending br. of occipital a.
(muscle br.)

Semispinalis capitis m.

Trapezius m.,
Splenius capitis m.

Fig. 13.6. The posterior neck region. The splenius capitis and trapezius muscle have been reflected medially.

The mastoid foramen is a large hole in the posterior border of the temporal bone. It transmits a mastoid emissary vein connecting the sigmoid sinus and a small meningeal branch of the occipital artery, the posterior meningeal artery, to the dura mater.

The semispinalis capitis muscle, situated deep to the splenius capitis and sternocleidomastoid muscle, attaches below to the upper thoracic and lower cervical vertebrae. The longissimus capitis muscle, situated deep to the splenius capitis

and sternocleidomastoid muscle, attaches above to the posterior margin of the mastoid process.

The greater occipital nerve ascends obliquely between the inferior oblique and the semispinalis capitis muscle. It pierces the semispinalis capitis and the trapezius muscles near their attachments to the occipital bone. It supplies the semispinalis capitis muscle, ascends with the occipital artery, and supplies the scalp as far forward as the vertex.

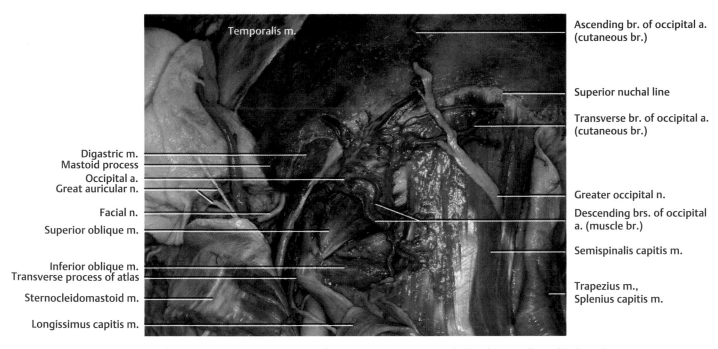

Temporalis m.

Ascending br. of occipital a. (cutaneous br.)

Superior nuchal line

Transverse br. of occipital a. (cutaneous br.)

Digastric m.
Mastoid process
Occipital a.
Great auricular n.

Facial n.

Superior oblique m.

Inferior oblique m.
Transverse process of atlas

Sternocleidomastoid m.

Longissimus capitis m.

Greater occipital n.

Descending brs. of occipital a. (muscle br.)

Semispinalis capitis m.

Trapezius m.,
Splenius capitis m.

Fig. 13.7. The posterior neck region. The longissimus capitis muscle has been reflected inferiorly.

The occipital artery arises from the posterior surface of the external carotid opposite the facial artery and runs posteriorly. At its origin, it is crossed by the hypoglossal nerve. On its way to the mastoid process, it crosses the internal carotid artery, the internal jugular vein, and the hypoglossal and spinal accessory nerves. It passes beneath the lower portion of the parotid gland. It runs horizontally backward through the occipital groove of the temporal bone, covered by all the muscles attached to the mastoid process: the sternocleidomastoid, splenius capitis, and the posterior belly of the digastric. It lies upon the superior oblique and semispinalis capitis muscle. The artery reaches the subcutaneous tissue by passing between the attachment of the trapezius and sternocleidomastoid muscle to the superior nuchal line.

The descending branch of occipital artery, the largest branch of the occipital, descends on the back of the neck and divides into a superficial and deep portion. The superficial portion runs beneath the splenius, giving off branches that pierce that muscle to supply the trapezius muscle. The deep portion runs down between the semispinalis capitis muscle and anastomoses with the vertebral artery.

The suboccipital muscles, located in the next layer, are a group of muscles situated deep to the splenius, semispinalis, and longissimus capitis in the suboccipital area. This group includes the superior oblique, which extends from the area lateral to the semispinalis capitis between the superior and inferior nuchal lines to the transverse process of the atlas; the inferior oblique, which extends from the spinous process and lamina of the axis to the transverse process of the atlas; the rectus capitis posterior major, which extends from and below the lateral part of the inferior nuchal line to the spine of the axis; and the rectus capitis posterior minor, which is situated medial to and is partially covered by the rectus capitis posterior major, and extends from the medial part and below the inferior nuchal line to the tubercle on the posterior arch of the atlas.

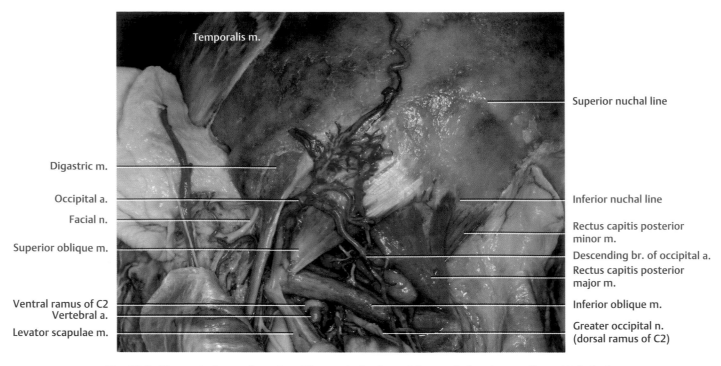

Fig. 13.8. The posterior neck region. The semispinalis capitis muscle has been reflected inferiorly.

The suboccipital triangle is a region bounded above and medially by the rectus capitis posterior major, above and laterally by the superior oblique, and below and laterally by the inferior oblique. The floor of the triangle is formed by the posterior atlanto-occipital membrane and the posterior arch of the atlas. The structures in the triangle are the terminal extradural segment of the vertebral artery and the first cervical nerve.

The C2 nerve emerges between the posterior arch of the atlas and the lamina of the axis where the spinal ganglion is located extradurally, medial to the inferior facet of C1 and the vertebral artery. The nerve divides into a large dorsal and a smaller ventral ramus. After passing below and supplying the inferior oblique muscle, the dorsal ramus divides into a large medial branch and a small lateral branch. It is the medial branch that forms the greater occipital nerve. The lateral branch sends filaments that innervate the splenius, longissimus, and semispinalis capitis, and is often joined by the corresponding branch from the C3 nerve. The C2 ventral ramus courses between the vertebral arches and transverse processes of the atlas and axis and behind the vertebral artery. Two branches of the C2 and C3 ventral rami, the lesser occipital and great auricular nerves, curve around the posterior border and ascend on the sternocleidomastoid muscle to supply the skin behind the ear.

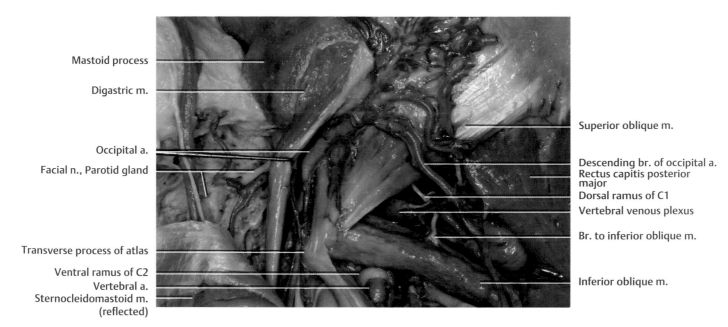

Mastoid process

Digastric m.

Superior oblique m.

Occipital a.

Facial n., Parotid gland

Descending br. of occipital a.
Rectus capitis posterior major
Dorsal ramus of C1
Vertebral venous plexus

Br. to inferior oblique m.

Transverse process of atlas

Ventral ramus of C2
Vertebral a.
Sternocleidomastoid m.
(reflected)

Inferior oblique m.

Fig. 13.9. The posterior neck region. The innervation to the muscles from dorsal ramus of C1 is shown.

The C1, C2, and C3 nerves divide into dorsal and ventral rami. The dorsal rami divide into medial and lateral branches that supply the skin and muscles of the posterior region of the neck. The C1 nerve, called the suboccipital nerve, leaves the vertebral canal between the occipital bone and atlas and has a dorsal ramus that is larger than the ventral ramus. The dorsal ramus courses between the posterior arch of the atlas and the vertebral artery to reach the suboccipital triangle, where it sends branches to the rectus capitis posterior major and minor, the superior and inferior oblique, and the semispinalis capitis. Occasionally, it has a cutaneous branch that accompanies the occipital artery to the scalp. The C1 ventral ramus courses between the posterior arch of the atlas and the vertebral artery and passes forward, lateral to the lateral mass of the atlas and medial to the vertebral artery, and supplies the rectus capitis lateralis.

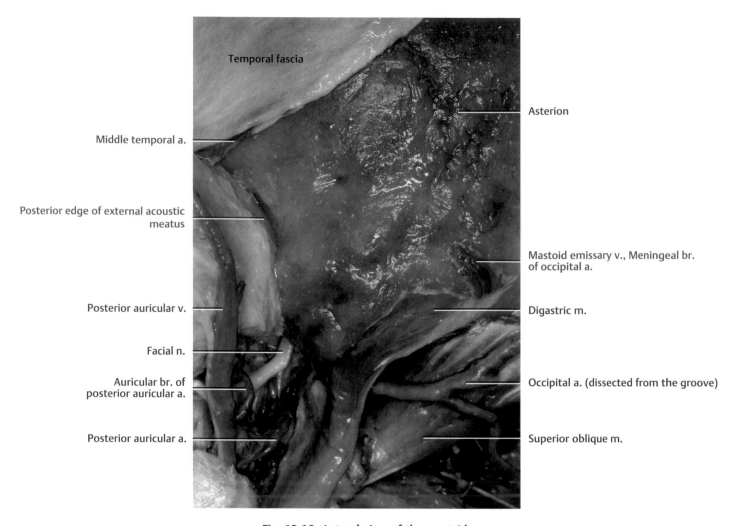

Fig. 13.10. Lateral view of the mastoid.

The posterior belly of the digastric muscle arises from the mastoid notch (digastric groove), which is on the inferior surface of the skull, medial to the mastoid process of the temporal bone. The posterior belly is supplied by the digastric branch of facial nerve. When the digastric muscle contracts, it acts to elevate the hyoid bone. If the hyoid bone is being held in place (by the infrahyoid muscles), it will tend to depress the mandible (open the mouth). The stylomastoid foramen is at the anterior end of the digastric notch.

The asterion, defined as the junction among the lambdoid, parietomastoid, and occipitomastoid sutures, is used as a landmark for the transverse-sigmoid sinus junction.

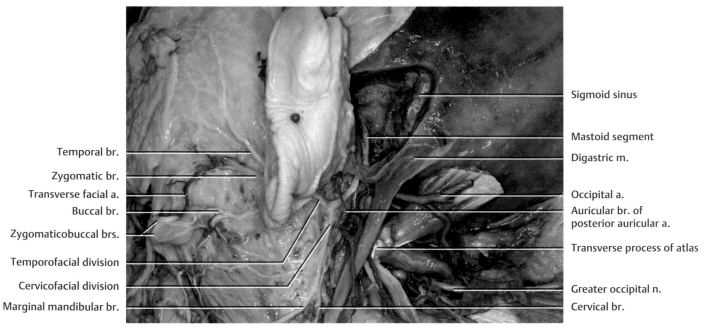

Fig. 13.11. The posterior neck region. The superficial lobe of the parotid gland has been removed and mastoidectomy has been completed.

After emerging from the base of the skull at the stylomastoid foramen, the facial nerve gains access to the face by passing through the substance of the parotid gland.

The branches in the face include the posterior auricular nerve, the nerve to the digastric and stylohyoid muscles, and the temporal, zygomatic, buccal, marginal mandibular, and cervical branches. The Inferior branches of the zygomatic branch usually form a zygomaticobuccal plexus with the buccal branches (see **Fig. 7.5**).

14 Lateral Neck Region

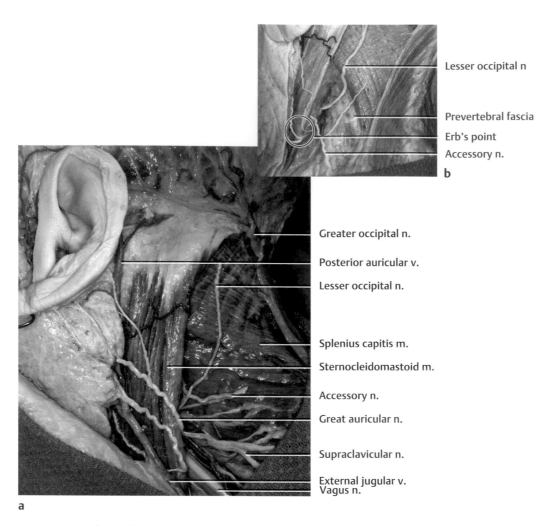

Lesser occipital n

Prevertebral fascia
Erb's point
Accessory n.

b

Greater occipital n.

Posterior auricular v.
Lesser occipital n.

Splenius capitis m.
Sternocleidomastoid m.

Accessory n.

Great auricular n.

Supraclavicular n.

External jugular v.
Vagus n.

a

Fig. 14.1a,b. (a) The lateral neck region. (b) Posterolateral view of the posterior triangle.

The cervical plexus is a plexus of the ventral rami of the first four cervical spinal nerves, which are located from C1 to C4 in the cervical segment in the neck. The branches of the cervical plexus emerge from the posterior triangle at Erb's point, a point midway on the posterior border of the sternocleidomastoid. The cervical plexus has two types of branches: cutaneous and muscular. The cutaneous branches are the lesser occipital nerve (C2), the great auricular nerve (C2, 3), the transverse cervical nerve (C2, 3), and the supraclavicular nerves (C3, 4). The muscular branches are the ansa cervicalis, phrenic, and segmental.

The lesser occipital nerve arises from the lateral branch of the ventral ramus of the second cervical nerve (C2). It curves around the accessory nerve and ascends along the posterior border of the sternocleidomastoid, where pierces the deep fascia near the cranium to supply the skin over the lateral scalp and posterior surface of the auricle. The great auricular and transverse cervical nerves only just enter the posterior triangle, turning sharply around the posterior border of the sternocleidomastoid muscle (Erb's point). The supraclavicular nerves emerge from beneath the sternocleidomastoid and pass across and down the posterior triangle toward the clavicle. The transverse cervical nerve supplies the skin anterolateral parts of the neck. The supraclavicular nerves supplies the skin over the pectoralis major and deltoideus and upper and posterior parts of the shoulder.

The prevertebral fascia is prolonged downward and laterally behind the carotid vessels and in front of the scaleni and forms a sheath for the brachial nerves and subclavian vessels in the posterior triangle of the neck.

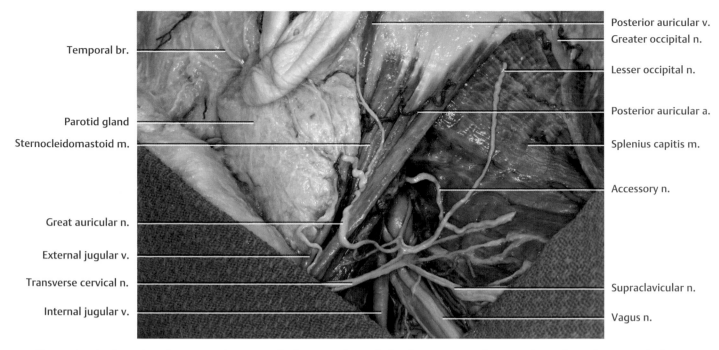

Temporal br.

Parotid gland

Sternocleidomastoid m.

Great auricular n.

External jugular v.

Transverse cervical n.

Internal jugular v.

Posterior auricular v.

Greater occipital n.

Lesser occipital n.

Posterior auricular a.

Splenius capitis m.

Accessory n.

Supraclavicular n.

Vagus n.

Fig. 14.2. The lateral neck region. The sternocleidomastoid muscle has been retracted anteriorly to show the cervical plexus.

The great auricular nerve is derived from the anterior rami of the C2 and C3 nerves. It appears at the posterior border of the sternocleidomastoid muscle and passes forward and upward across the muscle to reach the angle of the mandible on and beneath the parotid fascia. It supplies the skin overlying the mastoid process, lower part of the auricle, the parotid region, and the angle of the mandible. The great auricular nerve and sural nerve are the most commonly selected nerves for facial nerve grafting, but only 7 to 10 cm of the great auricular nerve can be harvested safely, which limits its use in extensive repairs. Disadvantages include a sensory deficit of the earlobe when using the great auricular nerve.

The accessory nerve also emerges from sternocleidomastoid muscle into the posterior triangle. The accessory nerve is found approximately 1 cm above Erb's point. It runs obliquely downward on the levator scapulae muscle to enter trapezius.

The external jugular vein lies on the lateral surface of the sternocleidomastoid muscle. It arises by the confluence of the posterior branch of the retromandibular vein and posterior auricular vein. It drains into the subclavian vein or internal jugular vein (see **Fig. 11.2**).

Index

Find 3D versions of all figures from
Atlas of the Facial Nerve and Related Structures
online at MediaCenter.thieme.com!

**Simply visit MediaCenter.thieme.com and, when prompted during the
registration process, enter the code below to get started today.**

255U-4C4A-LG4F-ALNN

	WINDOWS	MAC	TABLET
Recommended Browser(s)**	Microsoft Internet Explorer 8.0 or later, Firefox 3.x	Firefox 3.x, Safari 4.x	HTML5 mobile browser. iPad — Safari. Opera Mobile — Tablet PCs referred.
	** all browsers should have JavaScript enabled		
Flash Player Plug-in	Flash Player 9 or Higher* ** Mac users: ATI Rage 128 GPU does not support full-screen mode with hardware scaling*		Tablet PCs with Android OS support Flash 10.1
Minimum Hardware Configurations	Intel® Pentium® II 450 MHz, AMD Athlon™ 600 MHz or faster processor (or equivalent) 512 MB of RAM	PowerPC® G3 500 MHz or faster processor Intel Core™ Duo 1.33 GHz or faster processor 512MB of RAM	Minimum CPU powered at 800MHz 256MB DDR2 of RAM
Recommended for optimal usage experience	Monitor resolutions: • Normal (4:3) 1024×768 or Higher • Widescreen (16:9) 1280×720 or Higher • Widescreen (16:10) 1440×900 or Higher DSL/Cable internet connection at a minimum speed of 384.0 Kbps or faster WiFi 802.11 b/g preferred.		7-inch and 10-inch tablets on maximum resolution. WiFi connection is required.